Key Management Skills in Nursing
edited by
Roswyn A Brown and George Castledine

Managing the ethical process in research

by Marilyn Hammick

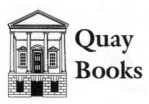

Quay
Books

Quay Books Division
Mark Allen Publishing Limited, Jesses Farm, Snow Hill
Dinton, Nr Salisbury, Wilts, SP3 5HN, United Kingdom

©Mark Allen Publishing Limited, 1996

British Library Cataloguing-in-Publication Data
A catalogue record for this book is available from the British Library

ISBN 1-85642-063-9

Printed in the UK by Biddles Ltd, Guildford and King's Lynn

Contents

Table of Figures

Dedication

This book is dedicated to my parents who set the scene for my personal ethical values. To my profession where examples abound for me of good practice in ethical health care and research. And to all the patients I have been privileged to care for who gave me a wealth of experience to enhance my learning.

Acknowledgements

I am indebted to Roswyn Brown for encouraging me to begin this book and for her timely, and always helpful, comments on the early drafts. My thanks also to Kumud Patel and Susan Pinder for their useful comments. I would also like acknowledge with thanks the sources of all the examples I have used. Without these, writing about the application of the principles of professionally and ethically responsible research would have been much more difficult. I am grateful for permission from John Wiley & Sons Ltd to make extensive reference to the ethical grid devised by Seedhouse and Lovett. Special thanks must go to my Father for his help with the early ideas for the illustrations, and to James for technical assistance. As always, I owe much to John who never ceases to give me the support I need, and to accept the time that my work takes from our life together.

Marilyn Hammick

Preface

This book on managing the ethical process is written for professionals from a wide range of disciplines whose job brings them into contact with people who need health or social care. They include nurses, the professions supplementary to medicine (chiropodists, dieticians, occupational therapists, physiotherapists, radiographers), social workers, probation officers, pharmacists, medical sociologists, clinical psychologists, counsellors etc. The list given here is not exhaustive and can include anyone whose professional practice may present ethical dilemmas, especially in relation to investigative work.

The emphasis throughout the book is on work done for research purposes. This often presents its own unique ethical issues and all proposals for research using human participants should undergo some form of ethical scrutiny.

The book aims both to inform and to guide. Some chapters discuss topics and issues related to ethically sound practice-based research. Other chapters aim to assist with three processes:

- *Personal ethical scrutiny of research*
- *Submittting a project for ethical clearance to either a research ethics committee or any other group with responsibility for ensuring that research participants are protected*
- *Enhancing the skills of members of ethics committees.*

Current developments in the caring professions which influence practice based research are reviewed. For novice researchers the book includes explanation and advice on some fundamental elements related both to ethics and investigative studies.

Throughout the book you will find words that are highlighted on their first appearance. This indicates that they are explained in the glossary. All the abbreviations and acronyms used are explained with their first use and listed at the end of the book. At the end of the book there is a reading and resources list which gives you some other sources of knowledge on the topic.

1
Health care, research and ethics: a tight bond

'I want to help people'

This is a common reply by applicants for health and psycho-social*
care pre-registration courses to the question, 'Why do you want to
be ...... a social worker (a physiotherapist, a nurse, a radiographer,
etc)'. In the first few years of learning and practising in these
professions the work revolves around direct care for people, much
of which is very personal.

The list of what we do is endless but it includes helping
people to:

- *Wash and relearn how to wash*
- *Move and adjust to physical disability*
- *Adapt to the psycho-social effects of an altered
  body image*

* Throughout the book reference is made to work
which involves helping people in some way. The author
recognises that such help is given in diverse ways by a variety
of professional and functional groups of workers. For
simplicity the generic word 'care' is used whenever possible.
Health care is also used frequently: this being the area with
which the author is most familiar. Social and psychological
and other forms of care can be substituted for health care in
most references.

- *Adjust to a new family lifestyle*
- *Accept treatments with acute short term effects.*

It means (amongst other things):

- *Holding their hand when words are insufficient*
- *Being there*
- *Knowing when not to be there*
- *Helping them to help themselves.*

At grassroots level in health and psycho-social care the practitioner works with real problems of real people facing trauma in their lives as well as seeking to provide support to the 'worried well' in health promotion activities. The way to help, care for, treat all of those in need, all of the time, in their best interests, inevitably produces dilemmas. Centrally directed policies and codes of conduct may guide professional practice: implementation by those at the 'coal face' often requires individual decision making and weighing up the rights and wrongs of what is to be done. From the beginning, practice means using personal moral standards to achieve an ethically sound outcome.

Career progression may change the way in which you use personal moral standards in your work. A move into management, working in a multi-disciplinary team, and becoming involved in research into practice all produce different problems but with the same need for ethically sound solutions.

Ethical decision making is part of the job at every level. Routine work puts us in contact with the people of today who need our help; research and development work ensures we consider the people of tomorrow. All this is done in the context of common principles that enable us to achieve our early ambition to help people. Two moral principles that help to form the ethical foundation of professional practice are:

- *Protection of the person receiving care*
- *Responsibility for giving care of the highest available quality.*

Protection of the patient** and offering quality care, as absolute standards, converge most naturally when practice is investigated. Both principles aim to ensure that, above all, the participants of research are protected and that:

> *'Concern for the interests of the subject ... always prevail(s) over the interests of science and society.'*
> (Declaration of Helsinki, 1.5) ***

In this book the topic of ethics in health care research is explored by considering the relationships between three elements:

1.   The professional practice of health care

2.   Investigation in health care practice

3.   Ethical principles in research

An indication of the links between these elements is shown in Figure 1.1. Each is briefly introduced in the next three sections of this chapter with more detailed consideration later.

1.1 Unpacking personal and professional ethics

The development of an ethical approach to how we examine in a rigorous way our practice(s) is stimulated by personal and professional knowledge and experience. As Figure 1.2 indicates there are unique features of each of these as well as areas of overlap.

We all carry with us our own ideas of what is right and what is wrong. The family, society and culture in which we grow and develop each have an impact on our moral standards. Our racial

---

**The word patient is used throughout this book to mean a person who is the recipient of care. In many care professions it may be more common to use the word client, or consumer or user. The word patient in many instances is synonymous with these and is used alone for simplicity.

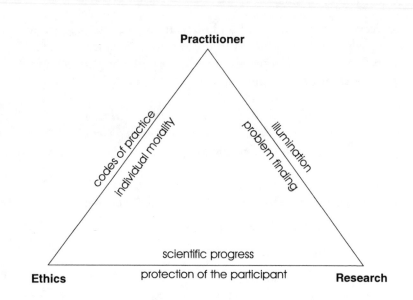

Figure 1.1 The health care, research and ethics triangle

origins and spiritual beliefs help to build for everyone of us a package of personal ethical values.

For all of us *'ethics originates in everyday life'* and should not be seen *'as a purely "academic" (sic) study.'* (Popkin & Stroll 1986, p.2)

With achievement of professional status we embrace codes of professional conduct to complement our personal bag of ethics. In figure 1.3 you can see examples taken from professional publications and codes of practice that relate to research.

***The Declaration of Helsinki was originally adopted by the 18th World Medical Assembly (WMA) in Helsinki, Finland, June 1964. It was amended by the 29th WMA, October 1975, the 35th WMA, October 1983 and the 41st WMA, September 1989.

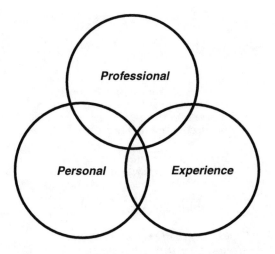

Figure 1.2 Personal, professional and experiential ethics

Other aspects covered in professional codes include:
- *Anonymising data*
- *Evaluation of practice*
- *A responsibility to publish results.*

Being professional means, amongst other things, making a commitment to keeping the standards embodied within professional codes. Deviance from them may result in removal of professional status and the right to practice.

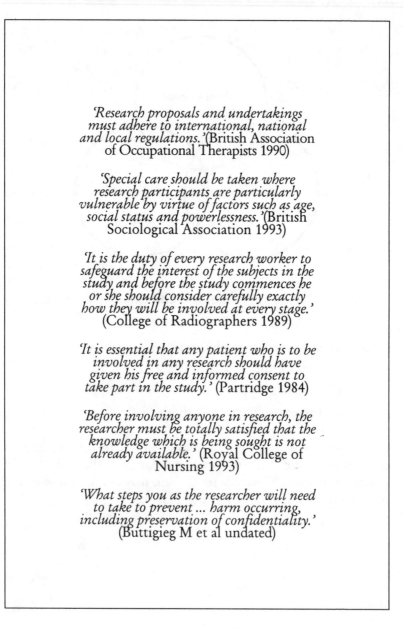

'Research proposals and undertakings must adhere to international, national and local regulations.'(British Association of Occupational Therapists 1990)

'Special care should be taken where research participants are particularly vulnerable by virtue of factors such as age, social status and powerlessness.'(British Sociological Association 1993)

'It is the duty of every research worker to safeguard the interest of the subjects in the study and before the study commences he or she should consider carefully exactly how they will be involved at every stage.' (College of Radiographers 1989)

'It is essential that any patient who is to be involved in any research should have given his free and informed consent to take part in the study.' (Partridge 1984)

'Before involving anyone in research, the researcher must be totally satisfied that the knowledge which is being sought is not already available.' (Royal College of Nursing 1993)

'What steps you as the researcher will need to take to prevent ... harm occurring, including preservation of confidentiality.' (Buttigieg M et al undated)

Figure 1.3 Research related codes of practice

The very nature of our work means we also gain the experience of coping with ethical dilemmas. Social and health care aim to support life both in quality and quantity whilst respecting as paramount the wishes of the patient. And this happens in an environment where resources are finite, the number of patients seems infinite and where history tells us that research is vital for progress. There are, of course, many other features of the health and social services, and those who need the help they offer, that introduce ethical issues into routine practice.

You will probably be able to think of times when you have considered the rights and wrongs of the way care is given:

- *In relation to an individual patient when the medical decision to continue with treatment seems at odds with allowing the patient to die with dignity*

- *When limited time and money are available and contracts decide a maximum age limit for patients to receive one type of therapy*

- *Listening to the debate about the acceptability of an organ donation system that requires people to opt out rather than to actively state they wish their kidneys, corneas etc to be used after their death.*

On these occasions we use heartfelt emotions, common sense, professional knowledge and past experience to reach decisions that are reasonable and fair. Put another way, the decisions reached feel morally sound and ethically just. If they don't feel like this we may be uncomfortable with the outcome. This may happen in situations that lead to clashes between professionals and their clients, where negotiation seems impossible and when we suspect our colleagues of malpractice or incompetence. These more negative experiences also contribute to the way we apply ethical values in health care.

With experience and knowledge we learn that ethical decision making is not a matter of absolute rights and wrongs.

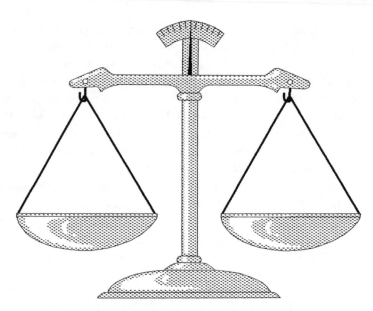

Figure 1.4 Balancing the issues

Between the perfect and supreme right at one end and the imperfect and undisputed wrong at the other is an inevitable grey area. Most of us will agree with actions assigned to each end of the spectrum. Put another way, the extremes are common to the majority. For example we would all acknowledge that the deliberate taking of human life is absolutely wrong.

But for most ethical dilemmas the answers come between the two ends, somewhere in the middle. And to complicate matters, because we are all unique individuals, with any one ethical dilemma, we will all probably be in a slightly different place between those two outermost points. You might like to try the following activity either by yourself, or with some colleagues if you feel comfortable sharing your views with them.

Think of some ethical dilemmas that arise in your work. Make a short list of them. It may be helpful to change each issue into a question. Decide the context of each one as far as you can. Are you considering it in relation to adults or children, that sort of thing?

For example, you might think about whether terminal and chronically ill patients have the right to decide for themselves that they should die i.e. the moral rights and wrongs of voluntary euthanasia. That probably has an impact on most care professionals and on all of us personally. The question to answer is, *'is euthanasia always unacceptable?'*.

Figure 1.4 shows scales which can measure from one extreme to the other, depending on what goes into the baskets on either side. Consider a scale like this for each of the dilemmas you are going to debate. Yes, you can have a debate with yourself. That is what you probably do quite often when making ethical decisions about caring for patients.

Think about the many aspects of your chosen ethical dilemma and put the different issues that arise in one basket or the other. Discuss how the issues move the pointer towards either end, or the other, of the scale. Consider why the position of the pointer changes with each individual's point of view, or with the different viewpoints you can think of for yourself.

You can also:

- *Compare your views with those of your colleagues*

- *Discuss how different, and how similar, the views you all have are?*

You will have realised by now that the value of this exercise is not simply identifying the place of the pointer on the scale. The benefit comes from participating in the debate on these sensitive and difficult issues. There are no definites in ethical decision making. It is a matter of moral reasoning to achieve a best possible outcome and this may differ with the circumstances and individual involved.

Moral reasoning is a question of balance and judgements based on personal and professional knowledge and experience. We each have a responsibility to learn how best to make these judgements and to ensure a balanced outcome in moral decision making. Nowhere is this more important than in investigative work which may not necessarily be for the direct benefit of the people who agree to take part in a study.

In the United Kingdom the responsibility for checking that research work is ethically sound rests with research ethics committees (REC). But, despite the existence of REC, researchers still have responsibilities for their work. To do this, as with other tasks health care practitioners and researchers 'need tools to be ethical' (Seedhouse 1988, p.90). In this way they are enabled to make moral decisions within a code of research ethics. Such a code could be described as:

> a set of principles which regulate and guide the behaviour of the researcher in their dealings with each other and with the participant of their studies (Popkin & Stroll 1986).

These principles are applicable in any situation where you are investigating or enquiring into professional practice. When:

| either | you are initiating a formal research project |
| or | you seek to find the answers to everyday questions by reflective practice. |

Ethics are the concern of everybody, each of us as professional practitioners, some of us as academic researchers, as we all strive to provide the very best care in the absolute interests of our patients.

1.2 Health care practice and research

Medical and health care professionals have long recognised the need for the development of methods of health care. A look back to the 19th Century shows us a classic example of a number of scientific discoveries which improved the health of the population.

Beginning in 1838, a series of events took place that transformed the impact of a number of infectious diseases on society:

1838 Chadwick wrote a report on the Sanitary Conditions of the Labouring Population which led to the establishment of a public health system (Watson 1969). This was instrumental in reducing mortality from infectious diseases such as cholera, typhoid and tuberculosis, by providing the clean water, food and air necessary for health.

1854 Snow confirmed the mode of transmission of cholera by comparative research into contamination of water supplies and this work led to eradication of this disease (Waters & Cliff 1983).

1860 Pasteur established the role of micro-organisms in transmissible diseases.

1880 Koch identified the organisms that caused cholera, typhoid, tuberculosis and other major infectious diseases (Duerden et al 1987).

1892 Haffkine developed a cholera vaccine which is now thought to be of limited efficiency(Duerden et al 1987). Vaccination does not prevent the spread of the disease and the recommended protection is to avoid the consumption of contaminated food and water.

1896 Wright discovered a vaccine (of killed suspensions of causative bacilli) for typhoid and it was widely used in the Boar War; but there was little evidence to support its effectiveness.

1929 Fleming discovered penicillin but not its therapeutic potential.

1941 Florey, Chain and associates commercially produced penicillin and made it available as a drug to treat infectious disease (Mandel et al 1985).

1947 Chloramphenicol was used to treat typhoid; other drugs now used include amoxycillin (Duerden et al 1987).

1954 Large scale trials in Yugoslavia showed the effectiveness of a heat-killed phenol-preserved typhoid vaccine (Duerden et al 1987).

1978 Taylor, investigating infection control procedures, identifies the poor handwashing techniques used by nurses; it is recommended that adequate handwashing will remove *'transient micro-organisms, picked up and shed.... during normal activities'* (Gould 1987, p.79).

1984 Ashworth proposes a *'hands and human beings'* approach to infection control rather than a *'rules, routines and rituals'* (Ashworth 1984 in Gould 1987, p.63).

The early epidemiological work of Chadwick and Snow had the major impact on the control of the predominant diseases of the time. Mortality rates from infectious diseases had started to fall rapidly prior to the introduction of drug related therapies. These enabled the patients still presenting with the disease to be cured. The introduction of a vaccination schedule further transformed the impact of most infectious diseases on late 20th century western societies. Research in the 1970's and 1980's returned to the basic principles of infection control but this time in relation to the nursing care of patients with infectious diseases in both general and isolation wards.

This brief historical look at the evolution of health care related to infectious diseases demonstrates the need for investigation into all aspects of the disease process and patient care. Different professionals, as individuals in the health care team, each make a unique contribution to total patient care. Similarly the motivation for research into new interventions and ways of working in health and social care settings is diverse. There is the natural curiosity of scientists. The increasingly recognised need to provide care that considers not only survival but also **quality of life outcomes**. Currently the ethos behind much research and development is the pursuit of value for money and efficiency.

For many years these motivators, but especially the drive to advance the technological base of medical science, have resulted in a great deal of medically orientated research. Most of this was, and still is, conducted within a **positivistic** framework, using **survival statistics** to measure success and measuring results by **mortality** and **morbidity**. This is very much the medically orientated assessment of an intervention. Rarely is the view of the patient taken into account.

Dominance of a medical model of health has meant less attention to the contribution to patient care by non-medical carers. But changes are happening within those professions who care for the patient as well as **about** the patient.

When we care for our patients we are concerned with:

- *The whole patient*
- *Their psycho-social well- being*
- *Their physical state of health*
- *Empowering them to help themselves*
- *The impact of treatment(s) now and in the future*
- *Enabling people to remain in control of their lives.*

This approach leans towards a social and person centred model of care. It opens up areas of development previously not well investigated and embraces all the disciplines that contribute to care.

An example of this is the joint development by physiotherapists, therapeutic radiographers and nurse specialists of an exercise schedule and advice clinic for women with breast cancer. The clinic is specifically for patients who are having radiotherapy, often following surgery. Such patients are at risk of developing post-surgical shoulder joint stiffness and upper limb lymphodeoma and need to know how to take care of their skin during and after radiation treatment. The side-effects of axillary surgery often prevents the patient maintaining the correct position for their post-operative radiotherapy and may lead to chronic mobility problems. At the clinic shared professional expertise has established a valuable service for patients that ensures accuracy and comfort during radiotherapy and helps to minimise long term debilitating side effects of treatment.

The introduction of the Patient'sCharter and increasing media interest in health provision are also contributing to the change. In some areas of health care, and for certain groups of patients there is a shift in the involvement of the patient in decision making in personal health care. A lot of patients now have enough knowledge about their disease and its management to allow them to make truly informed decisions about treatment alternatives and whether or not they wish to participate in research studies. Many women with breast cancer come into this group with health education programmes, self-help groups and breast care nurse specialists all providing advice, information and support.

Others may feel less well informed and less confident about asking questions about what is happening to them. People from ethnic minority groups and elderly men are but two examples of those who may need support and advocacy during the process of giving informed consent. Acting as a **patient advocate** and/or **interpreter** to patients is yet another research role for the professional.

The example of joint developments such as sanitation, anti-biotic therapy, vaccination and infection control in hospitals shows how diverse changes lead to improvements in managing disease and preventing ill-health. A century and a half after Chadwick it is now widely accepted that all health professionals have a responsibility to introduce only those new methods of care that have been rigorously investigated.

There is also the need for continuous evaluation of current working practices. Because of the very nature of health care work, most studies will be on people, or with people related data. This type of work requires checks and balances to ensure that the participants of research are protected at all times. This procedure is known as ethical scrutiny. It is currently done by health care professionals either as members of REC or other research vetting groups. Health care and services researchers are responsible for

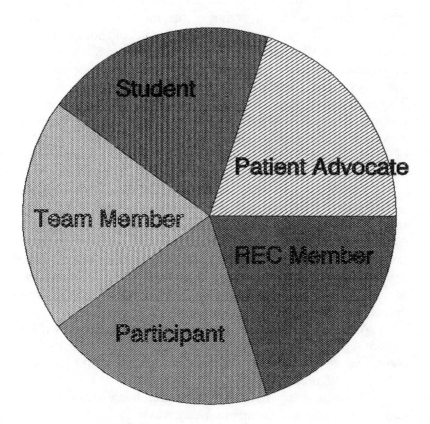

Figure 1.5 Involvement in research

putting their work forward for ethical scrutiny. But before that they need to personally check their proposals. The practitioner-researcher has a responsibility to ensure that their investigative work is done within the same moral boundaries that ɔutine work. Some knowledge of research ethics and the pːⱅ..... of ethical scrutiny will help you to do this.

1.3 Research ethics

The focus on health care in the previous sections, rather than medical care, respects the value of the multi-disciplinary team approach. Different disciplines working collaboratively to improve the quality and quantity of life of patients. But it is to the term medical ethics we must turn for the first references to the need to protect participants of research. As long ago as 1803 Thomas Percival suggested peer discussion of new ideas for this purpose. The end of World War 2 saw international attempts to prevent atrocities being committed against human life in the name of medical research. At this time, in particular, the importance of informed consent was stressed.

The topic of informed consent is one of the dominant issues at meetings of REC today. A recent study of several REC found that, *'the main concerns that ... members referred to as "ethical" (sic) were largely relating to consent'*(Neuberger 1992, p.43). In a detailed case study on one REC, informed consent was found to be the most regular issue discussed at meetings (Hammick 1993). Guidelines on research ethics by public, professional and commercial organisations devote a lot of space to consent issues.

A recent Government publication recommends that,'written consent should be required for all research' and 'for therapeutic research consent should be recorded in the patient's medical records' (Department of Health 1991, p.12).

Ensuring that participants of research freely give informed consent to their involvement in any study is fundamental to carrying out ethically sound research. This topic is looked at in detail in chapter seven. In particular, guidance on writing patient information sheets (PIS) that are ethically sound is included. It is the wording of these that often fails to meet the standards of those who are responsible for ethical scrutiny.

Throughout their professional lives health care practitioners may take different roles within the research process. In each of these different ethical issues may arise. The ethical dilemmas in any situation depend upon many things. The people involved, their personal morality, the need to respect the autonomy of each individual; all these contribute to the uniqueness of any situation. The state of current knowledge on a topic is also a powerful influence on the process of finding **the best possible under the circumstances** answer where problems are related to the morality of a situation.

The different ways you may be involved in research work are shown in Figure 1.5.

Each of the roles shown in Figure 1.5 has its individual features and each one overlaps with some of the others.

For example informed consent is a feature in the following situations:

- *You may be asked to act solely as patient advocate when informed consent is sought from people asked to enter a multi-centred clinical trial or a sociological survey of patients attitudes*

- *In a study where you are the only person doing the work, for perhaps a masters degree course, it is your responsibility to obtain informed consent from potential participants*

- *As part of a research team you will need to agree with colleagues on the process of how to obtain the consent of participants in a way that is as free as possible from any bias by each member of the team*

- *A colleague asks you to participate in a study and you need to be assured of just what you are consenting to*

- *As a member of an ethics committee you are responsible for reviewing the way the researchers plan to obtain informed consent from potential participants.*

Whatever your role an understanding of the issues surrounding the process of obtaining informed consent will be helpful.

Accepting and evaluating the practicalities of the research process within an ethical framework is vital and these concern you when:

- *As a principal investigator you are accountable for a resource intensive project and responsible for securing funding to prevent money from the service budget being misdirected into research work*

- *As patient advocate you are responsible for ensuring that individualised care of the highest quality is still available for non-participants of the study*

- *As part of a faculty team that scrutinises proposals to allocate funding for research involving people you will have a responsibility to ensure that the researchers are able to carry out the work and use the money given to them wisely.*

Whatever your role in a project the research methods used will vary depending upon the scientific basis of the investigative work. This, in turn, may influence the ethical principals that need consideration. In relation to the research process scientific and ethical principles are closely linked. The need to *'conform to generally accepted scientific principles'* is the first basic principle of biomedical research involving human subjects (Declaration of Helsinki, 1.1). In health and social care a broad spectrum of the natural and the human sciences are studied using a variety of research methodologies. You may have been involved in studies which have used different methods of collecting information and distinct ways of analysing data.

The role you take in the research process and the research methods and tools you use may vary. Whatever the differences you have a responsibility to ensure that ethical principals are maintained. Involvement in health care research requires an ethical framework to guide your opinion and judgements.

In the next chapter the context and need for ethically based research into all aspects of health care work is looked at in detail. You will probably be able to identify with some of the situations discussed. Following this there are five chapters which aim to provide you with information and guidance on two separate but overlapping processes of ethical scrutiny.

Chapters three and four take a detailed look at research ethics. They aim to assist with ways that you, as an individual researcher, can ethically evaluate all the aspects of your research from proposal, through methodology, to writing the report. Chapters five and six consider the process of ethical scrutiny by committees responsible for protecting people as potential participants. Advice on how to successfully apply for ethical clearance is given in relation to completing the paperwork and being interviewed. Chapter seven discusses some issues surrounding informed consent and preparation of PIS to accompany consent forms.

2
Emergence of new research paradigms

Where has the drive to research into methods of caring for patients come from?

What has brought about the rapid increase in nursing research?

Who is responsible for the emergence of research to underpin the practice of radiography?

Three searching questions which feature just two of the rapidly developing research based health care disciplines. Other professions, for example physiotherapy and speech therapy, are similarly strengthening their research foundation. Within these different disciplines new methods of practice based care are emerging as the result of careful and systematic investigation.

Studies using a variety of methods across a spectrum of health and social sciences are regular features of the research work in many hospitals and primary care settings. The need to gain expertise and experience in the use of data collection tools and analytical techniques is recognised. Fundamental to these changes is the learning of skills of ethical evaluation of research proposals.

2.1 Expansion of research and graduate status

The move toward all graduate entry for the professions supplementary to medicine (PSMs), and the increase in the numbers of nurses with graduate qualifications, has influenced the rapid expansion in research work in these health care disciplines. The development of under- and post-graduate courses has been accompanied by recognition of the need for all care practitioners to develop research based practices. Research into both routine and potential new methods of care strengthens the link between theory and practice. Figure 2.1 shows how both these essential parts of education programmes and professional practice interact with the other. As Lenin reminds us, *'theory without practice is barren but practice without theory is blind'.**

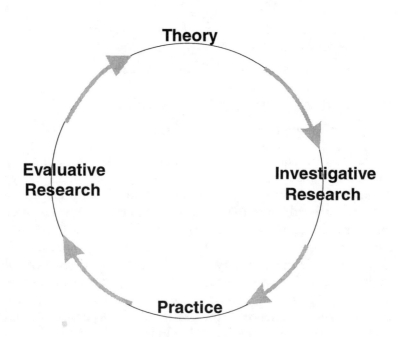

Figure 2.1 Research, theory and practice

*This quote was attributed to Lenin in an informal conversation between the author and colleagues. All attempts to verify the source and to date the quote have failed. It is, therefore, recognised that the words may, or may not, have been first used by Lenin.

A great deal of health care practice is based upon tradition (with and without theory) rather than research (Thompson et al 1988). But today's practitioners are less accepting of this legacy than their predecessors. There is wide acknowledgment that **empirical** studies have much to contribute to the evaluation of the entire service offered to patients. Professional responsibility includes recognising that:

> *'it is unethical for the profession to fail to do*
> *research because this deprives present and future*
> *patients of the possibility of more informed and*
> *better treatment as well as the (more distant)*
> *prospect of the prevention of... disorder'* (College
> of Psychiatrists 1990, p.48).

Continuation of a total health care service is also dependant upon maintaining the quality of practitioner education. Practice based education rapidly becomes valueless if what is practised is not continuously evaluated. Completion of the move of schools of nursing, radiography, physiotherapy etc into higher education has the potential to widen the gap between theory and practice. In many cases the recent changes of responsibility for nursing and PSMs education programmes have meant geographical relocation away from hospital sites. This separation of the clinical and academic education base must not be accompanied by separation of clinical and school based elements of health care curricula. The integration of teaching and research will ensure *'competence and efficiency ... and the most effective and cost-efficient care for ... patients,'*(Thompson et al 1988, p.76).

2.2 Expansion of research into fresh fields

With the ever increasing complexity of medical technology, the establishment of the internal market into the National Health Service (NHS) and the potential introduction of concepts such as Quality Adjusted Life Years (QALYs), future research needs to expand into areas previously untouched. A 1988 report from the

- *The impact of published authoritative research on purchasing and clinical practice*[1]
- *Aspects of screening for hearing loss in the over-75 age group*[1]
- *Teenage pregnancy*[1]
- *Dental health needs of ethnic minorities*[1]
- *The value of integrating quality of life data and data on costs in the measurements of outcomes in prevention, treatment and care of cancer patients and their carers*[2]
- *The psychosocial needs of under-served groups (the elderly, children, ethnic minorities) and of carers, both families and professionals*[2]

Source: advertisements by[1]South East Thames Regional Health Authority and [2]South and West Regional Health Authority (1994)

Figure 2.2 Invitations to research

King's Fund entitled 'The Nation's Health', and the more recent Department of Health strategy document 'The Health of the Nation' (1992), both comment about the need for the promotion of public health to be supported by research and development. Locally each health region is inviting tenders for research into specified topics. Figure 2.2 demonstrates the kind of areas that are currently attracting research funding and thus invitations to tender for the research work.

These, and others mentioned in the NHS Research & Development Strategy document, need a multi-disciplinary research team if holistic care is to become practice rather than rhetoric.

We are also seeing the advent of health services research or *'the identification of the health care needs of communities and the study of the provision, effectiveness and use of health services,'*(Medical Research definition in Clarke & Kurinczuk 1992, p. 1675).

The paper:

Marcus A C[1], Cella D[2], Sedlacek S[3], Crawford E D[4], Crane L A[5], Garrett K[6], Quigel C[7], Gonin R[8] (1993) Psychosocial counselling of cancer patients by telephone: a brief note on patient acceptance of an outcall strategy. *Psycho-Oncology* vol. 2: 209-214

The researchers:

[1]Director of Public health research, Cancer research centre; [2]Director of Psychosocial oncology, Cancer institute; [3]Medical oncologist; [4]Professor of urology, University health sciences centre; [5] Behavioural scientist and [6]Programme co-ordinator, Cancer research centre; [7] Clinical research nurse, University health sciences centre, [8]Bio-statistician, Cancer institute and School of public health.

Figure 2.3 Multi-disciplinary research in cancer care

Health services research will undoubtedly benefit from a multi-disciplinary research approach that draws investigators from diverse fields of health care.

Figure 2.3 highlights the different disciplines that worked together in a well focused study to develop a speciality service. The research reported in this particular paper investigated the response of patients to a telephone psycho-social counselling service. It asked potential service users what they thought. The study is a good example of how *qualitative* and *quantitative* data collection tools (interview and survey by closed questions) can complement each other to further knowledge. **Do try to read it.**

2.3 Practice based research and evaluation

The increase in the number of investigative studies into the practice of every health care discipline is a welcome development. Many of these form an integral part of the academic context of the profession. Honours and masters degree programmes require that students experience the research process. They aim to equip the learner with the knowledge and skills to enquire deeply into a selected topic. To examine it in detail. This is often the introduction for many practitioners to the research process. Many of you will be familiar with it as a step along the way towards future individual and team contributions to research based care.

Compatibility between levels of academic study and the students experience of research is vital. Research in the curriculum needs to allow for progression in both the learning of how to do research and the acquisition of positive values about the role of research in practice. This may be achieved within the following framework:

Diploma level	an appreciation of research
Honours degree	a pilot study or literature based individual project
Masters degree	a small scale study using observation or experiment that contributes to the body of knowledge

| Doctoral study | original, investigative work that makes a major contribution to the body of knowledge and may alter practice |

It is important that studies are not only done as part of pre- and post-registration degree courses but as part of the routine work of practitioners and academics. This is not to devalue the contribution made by research done as part of assessment for university and professional award courses. Students at first and second degree level, and those that proceed to a doctorate, will all contribute to the body of knowledge. They will also take research experience and expertise into their clinical workplace. But the value of research within academic programmes is only fully realised when accompanied by a commitment to research within practice. In this way we can be sure that only those health care techniques that have been scientifically investigated to prove their efficacy are used.

Many of you reading this book may be doing research for the first time. Alternatively, you may have the experience of a relatively small individual piece of investigative work behind you and now feel confident to do further research as part of practice related work. Whatever the case, it is likely that the topic of investigation has come from your professional practice. This is, of course, the way forward.

Each discipline has the unique knowledge of how to develop its own practice. Staff with the potential for identifying topics that need investigation and offer the promise of improving care include:

- *Policy makers*
- *General and professional managers*
- *Practitioners at the patient face.*

Within each discipline the methods of investigation will have features distinctive of the way they deliver care and features which are common to research methods used by other care professionals. We then see the emergence of discipline specific **paradigms** that shape the research done on ideas and issues originating from within each of the care professions. This research should be motivated only by the demand for further knowledge and understanding, and not constrained in any way.

Constraint may appear in many guises:

- *The need to negotiate ethical scrutiny can influence the topic of research proposals, especially for the novice investigator*
- *Socialisation by the paradigms of other related disciplines.*

Socialisation or the acquisition of the scope and means of investigative work from other care professionals with established research paradigms, is a trap to be avoided. It is vital that individual professional paradigms develop internally, as the result of intra-disciplinary pressure. Modelling new work on current paradigms may not serve the best interests of patients where total care is the required outcome.

In some areas of health care nurses and other health practitioners have taken the role (often informally) of research assistants to medical colleagues. This contribution, whilst valuable experience, can subordinate the role of non-medical practitioner/researchers. All practitioners and professions at the threshold of developing a research practice need advice, guidance and co-operation, and should be mindful of the opportunity to learn from the experience of others. But finally we have to be convincing as research based practitioners in our own right. Negotiating ethical clearance and satisfying a REC is part of the process of assuring that the value of our investigative work is recognised by colleagues in all the other disciplines of health care.

Your research work may be theoretical or empirical, a piece of qualitative or quantitative research, or an extensive literary review . Whatever it is, if it is ethically sound, it will be of value. Of value for the content and for encouraging the so very essential spirit of enquiry into practice. The findings may initiate a change in practice, or lead to further work as all good research should. Importantly, though, the researcher will have experienced the process of questioning practice and the value of reflecting on practice.

Research which opens up unsuspected gaps in knowledge and which identifies further problems provides the material for future solutions. Advances in practice emerge by this dual system of identifying gaps or finding problems and filling gaps or solving problems. Problem finding is creative and original in comparison to problem solving which is routine and aims at conclusive evidence or proof. Both are essential to the development of any scientific discipline, whether a natural or applied health care science. Once this absolutely vital first step of identifying what needs to be investigated is done the researcher can begin to decide how to carry out the study.

2.4 Different methods of research: similar ethical issues

How the scientific inquiry proceeds is determined by the very nature of the study. The natural sciences are more likely to be brought to the clinical setting after preliminary laboratory work. This is the more orthodox approach with an:

> '*apparatus of experimental method,*
> *quasi-experimental method,* **statistical**
> **significance,** *dependant and independent*
> **variables,** *and so on'* (Reason & Rowan 1981,
> p.xiii).

The human sciences demand a different approach. There is greater use of qualitative methods. The **phenomenological** and **ethnographic** approaches are common. Case studies are frequently done. Data collection tools are different. Observation and **interviews** are used as ways of providing information that is detailed and usually related to few rather than many participants. In contrast the **double blind clinical trial,** using quantitative techniques and providing sound and generalisable data, dominates research into new medical interventions.

A different approach to the investigation does not exclude it from the label of scientific inquiry. All research methods seek to be either *'descriptive (or) theoretical'* and these are aspects of scientific activity (Von Wright 1978, p.11). A human or social science study may be imaginative and creative, concerned with interpretation. A natural scientific study is likely to be more defined, with stated procedures and a clear direction from the early stages of the study. Both have elements of serendipity and rigour though perhaps in differing amounts. In other words throughout the research process there may be discovery by chance, unplanned and unexpected alongside and within the logical structure and exacting nature of the research design. Both are essential to the continued development of health care procedures. Rowan (1981, p.40) suggests that advances in science happen when *'scientists of widely different persuasions'* thrust *'their opposing conceptions and commitments at each other'.*

The diverse ways in which care is given to patients in the different settings of the health service means that equally diverse research methods will be used. We are currently seeing the emergence of new ways of investigating how to care for the patient as a physical and psychosocial whole person. Social science research tools are proposed as valuable within the health care sciences. We need to be aware of the resistance within the scientific community of the health service to different research approaches. Nursing research (and other human science studies) *'may be disvalued'* , seen as *'soft science or even unscientific'* (Hunt 1992, p.5).

Data from a case study of a REC indicates conflict related to so-called simple protocols, which was how non-medical studies tended to be seen (Hammick 1993). They sometimes received a lot of attention because they were so easily understood. Alternatively they were dismissed because of their simplicity in contrast to the more complex studies with high costs, using complex therapies that may be a risk to life. Either way non-medical studies using social science methodologies may not be taken seriously.

A REC used to dealing with natural science methods can have difficulty in recognising the scientific worth of human or social science studies. One solution is fair representation of the different sciences within the membership of these committees. And researchers submitting projects to REC need to ensure that their proposals are ethically sound. The intervention may be different in a non-medical study but it still impacts upon the life of the patient who consents to be a participant.

Whether it is a thought provoking semi-structured interview, extra blood tests or the side-effects of new drugs we need to evaluate that impact from an ethical viewpoint. The concept of invasiveness is not limited to breaching the physical barrier of research participants, i.e. to invading their body. It must also be recognised as trespassing in other, perhaps more concealed areas, such as their psychological well-being and social life.

2.5 Wider issues: publication and business ethics

Completing a piece of research, reaching conclusions and making recommendations, is an important step on the way to persuading others of its value. The College of Radiographers 1994 Strategy for Research highlights that, *'It is a fact that research does not "exist" (sic) unless it is published.'* If you want to convince those who control resources that an aspect of routine practice needs changing, or that new methods of care are needed, you need to bring your work to the attention of other people. You can do this by:

either
- giving presentations about your work (Figure 2.4)

or
- making written reports available (Figure 2.4)

Your research report needs to be read widely, not only by the supervisor and assessor at the university, or colleagues who helped you with the project. For different readers you may need to adapt your report; leaving in the major points of interest to the particular

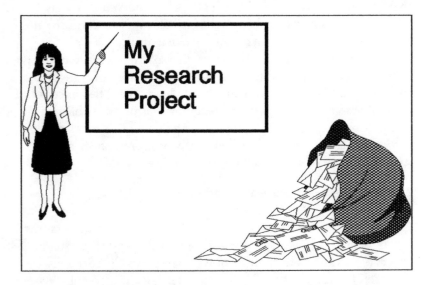

Figure 2.4 Presenting and distributing your research

reader and omitting certain sections. You should be sensitive to issues within your findings that may rock the boat, either professionally or politically; remember that the ethical approach includes respect for everyone's rights. In a given circumstance it might be appropriate for you to only submit the abstract. In this way there is some chance of the new ideas born out of your research becoming reality.

Publication in a reputable journal is vital. Without this your work may remain on the library shelf, or in the bottom drawer of the desk. The need for ethical work not to waste resources, whether financial or time and effort by professionals and the participants, is examined later. The important issue here is to ensure that your report is accepted for publication. The majority of health care journals require evidence of ethical clearance for studies involving people. Yet another reason for you to understand the process of ethical scrutiny. Don't forget to include in your research report that permission to proceed with a study was given by the appropriate REC.

Another way of bringing your work to the attention of a wider audience is by talking about it. Offer to speak at your hospitals' lunchtime seminar and to talk at a professional association meeting. Confidentiality and anonymity are ethical issues that need careful consideration when you discuss your research outside of the setting in which it took place. It is your responsibility to ensure that the location and personnel involved in your research cannot be identified. The same concerns can arise if the report of the investigation is available for reading by people other than those who participated and supported the work.

This, of course, happens with research done for a university based course. The final bound documents become part of the academic library, accessible to other students and staff for many years. The need to ensure that participants involved in your research remain anonymous, and individual data confidential to the researcher only is a fundamental principal of ethically sound research. What may be more difficult is the need to respect the organisation, or parts of the organisation investigated.

The researcher has a duty to prevent the name and location of any group, organisation or company who agree to take part in a study from becoming public knowledge. Apart from not making open references we also should be aware of how easy it can be for others to deduce from our work where the study took place.

The advent of a business environment in the NHS means competition. This competitive drive may open up an unhealthy potential for data on a particular organisation to be useful to someone else in the same market. Employees need to be aware of maintaining confidentiality about operational and financial policies. A breach of that trust could curtail the types of investigations permitted; it could put an unwanted brake on the rights of the professional to explore and evaluate all aspects of health care practice.

This chapter has highlighted the ethical and scientific maze to be negotiated by researchers into health care services and methods. The more you know about that maze the easier it will be to successfully make your way through it. The best way to learn is, of course, by experience. But before you do that read on. The next few chapters aim to make that experience as interesting and as enjoyable as possible.

3
Research ethics: philosophy and principles

Philosophy may be defined as:

> *'the use of reason and argument in seeking truth and knowledge'* (Concise Oxford Dictionary 1990)

where this leads to a set of beliefs. **Principles** are fundamental laws and rules that form a basis to reason and act from. This chapter considers the philosophies and principles of ethical research in different ways, putting them together in an algorithm or set of rules that can be used for assessing the ethical nature of investigative work. The algorithm is called a Research Ethics Wheel (REW) and is modelled on a grid devised to assist with decision-making processes in clinical practice (Seedhouse & Lovett 1992).

The original grid *'enable(s)the clinician to justify his solution to himself, or to other people'* (Seedhouse & Lovett 1992, p. 21). It has elements in common with, and relevant to, research ethics. The REW has been adapted to reflect the purpose and process of the ethical scrutiny of research proposals, imitating the original grid but also deviating from it, making the segments pertinent to investigative work. It uses empirical evidence from studies on REC as its building blocks and presents a whole pattern to guide the researcher. The REW aims to help the researcher to apply the process of moral reasoning to a proposal for investigative work i.e. to undertake ethical self-scrutiny.

As researchers we are obliged to assess the ethics of studies involving patients or their data; it would be unethical merely to rely on the formal procedure for ethical scrutiny. As with all the other tasks that make up the complex process of research the researcher needs to know something about the factors that are considered in the process of moral reasoning. Seedhouse (1988, p.90) refers to this in a similar way by his assertion that:

> *'health workers need to know the basic content of and difficulties with the various theories of ethics, and they need to be aware of the different principles for action that follow from the various theories'.*

With knowledge of the factors the practitioner is better able to make moral decisions within a code of research ethics. Such a code has an underlying philosophy and set of principles which direct and guide the behaviour of the researcher in their dealings with each other and with the participants of their studies.

3.1 The Research Ethics Wheel

The Wheel is divided into four quarters, each with four segments. Each segment is designed to provoke thought and reason during ethical self-scrutiny of a research proposal. Figure 3.1 shows the complete REW. In later sections each quarter is dissected out and the segments are disassociated. The pattern is similar to that used by Seedhouse in his original Ethical Grid. Within each quarter, different aspects of moral reasoning are shown but the divisions are there for convenience and the REW is a flexible tool. The segments have ethical issues in common and should not be seen in isolation from each other.

Each quarter of the Wheel focuses on four fundamental ingredients for moral reasoning through which relevant and necessary portions can be weighed up and considered. The process involves selecting the portions that will help to achieve an effective judgment about the ethics of a research proposal. Such a judgement will feel comfortable and morally sound to the researcher. No one ingredient is more important than any of the others. In given situations the recipe for ethical decision making may exclude one or more of them. To help in the ethically sound decision making

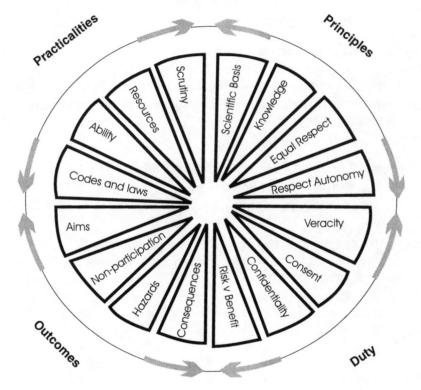

Figure 3.1 The Research Ethics Wheel

process the issues in several of the segments form part of the deliberation.

Four fundamental aspects of research work underline each quarter, these are the:

- **Principles** *of research using people*
- **Duties** *of a researcher*
- **Nature** *of the outcome of the research*
- **Practicalities** *of the research process.*

3.2 Principles of ethical research

The first quarter of the REW illustrates the principles behind research with people as participants. These fundamental principles are that research should:

- *Have a scientific basis*
- *Improve knowledge and understanding*
- *Respect all people equally*
- *Respect the autonomy of people.*

The four segments in Figure 3.2 show the principles which are now explored in detail to assist with the process of reasoning about the ethics of a research proposal.

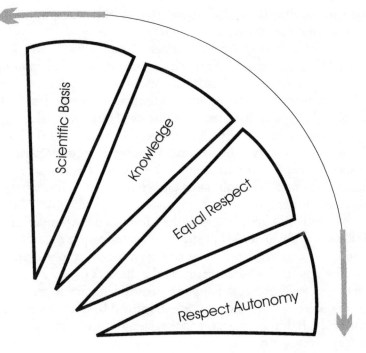

Figure 3.2 Principles of Ethical Research

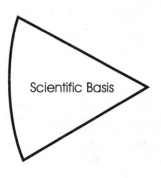

The need to do investigative work in a scientific manner and to *'conform to generally accepted scientific principles'* is the first basic principle of biomedical research involving human subjects (Declaration of Helsinki, 1.1). There is controversy about what constitutes scientific research and a tendency to regard investigations into the natural sciences by traditional or orthodox methods as more worthy of that label than those done within disciplines of the human or social sciences.

Not only is this view threatening to the vital and valuable research carried out in these sciences but it may lead to either a complacent, or a confrontational, attitude towards certain studies. This, in turn, leads to minimal attention to the ethics of these studies. The researcher needs to be aware of this potential difficulty when approaching a REC. It is important to understand why, and be ready to justify why, ethical scrutiny is as important for a research proposal in the human sciences as it is for one in the natural sciences. The following paragraphs seek to illuminate this topic further.

Study in a broad range of the natural and the human sciences is needed to enhance the holistic care of those people needing health and social care services. To be of use all investigations eventually require application, to humans, of the theories they seek to prove or disprove. Whether the applied scientific inquiry is preceded by pure experimentation or not is determined by the very nature of the study. It differs according to the scientific discipline of the topic under investigation.

The human sciences often demand a more unorthodox approach, described as *'objectively subjective'* and a *'synthesis of naive inquiry and orthodox research,'* (Reason & Rowan 1981, p. xiii).

An alternative way of seeing these two types of research is to view the researchers as different types of scientist:

- *The analytical with a basic drive towards certainty, concerned with 'precision, accuracy and reliability'*

- *The conceptual, concerned with imagination, speculation and with a style and outlook which aims to 'further the development of human growth, awareness and general welfare' either in general or in particular (Reason 1981, pp.45-50).*

Health care research embraces the natural and human sciences and thus many different enquiry systems and approaches to objectivity, validity and truth (Rowan 1981).

These are very good reasons for REC to support and scrutinise research from all the sciences. Equally, researchers, investigating topics in the human and social sciences, need to be ready to:

- *Defend the scientific principles of their investigative work*

- *Guard against any disregard by others of the need for ethical scrutiny of their research proposals.*

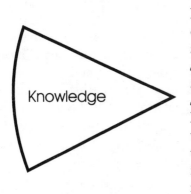

The Declaration of Helsinki states that the purpose of biomedical research is *'to improve diagnostic, therapeutic and prophylactic procedures and the understanding of the aetiology and pathogenesis of disease.'* The REW includes the requirement to improve knowledge and understanding, and to alert the researcher to the responsibility not to do investigative work for the sake of the work alone. It is unethical to use resources (time, money etc) and to involve other people (colleagues and potential participants) in work that will not add to the body of knowledge within a particular scientific discipline.

This is not to say that investigations may not be repeated. Many topics benefit from further enquiry and it is rare that one study alone discovers all there is to know about a topic. There are a number of ways in which one investigation may differ from another and may yield extra knowledge.

These include:

- *Using a different setting to ascertain the influence of location on the results*
- *Studying a different group of participants by increasing the age range of the sample*
- *Increasing the sample size to obtain more quantitative data*
- *Decreasing the sample size to obtain more qualitative data*
- *Investigating the same issues in a different cultural group.*

The list given above is not endless and indicates that the researcher rarely needs to feel constrained about the choice of topic to investigate. This is especially so with practice-based research since it is highly unlikely that the factors associated with one clinical practice setting will be exactly the same as any other.

However, the researcher is acting against ethical principles if their work does not aim to find out anything that is not already known. This includes:

- *Doing a thorough review of the literature on a topic before proceeding with investigative work*
- *Not using elderly books and journal articles which may generate out-of-date material and be misleading as to the current state of knowledge on a topic.*

This preparatory work gives a sound background to the proposed work and often highlights the present gaps in knowledge about a topic. Searching the literature and probing other sources of knowledge on a topic is an effective way of formulating a research proposal. The search provides what is already known and the presently unanswered questions; the proposal aims to fill in the gap between these two, or at least some of it!

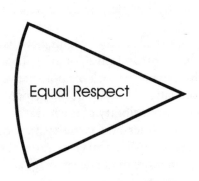

Equal Respect

Another feature of the first quarter of the REW is that all persons should be respected equally, not only because of what they can do but also because of what they are (Seedhouse 1988). Every effort must be made at each stage of the research process to ensure that every potential and actual participant is treated the same.

It is the researcher's responsibility to ensure that there is no discrimination on the grounds of:

- *Education and intellectual attainment*
- *Physical and mental ability*
- *Race*
- *Ethnicity and cultural background*
- *Religion*
- *Age*
- *Gender and sexual orientation.*

Upholding this principle during the process of ethical research means:

- *Respect for people who do not wish to be included because the study may conflict with their beliefs and values*
- *Respect for people who would wish to participate but who may be or feel excluded because of their culture, age, gender, language skills etc.*

Application of this principle involves an appreciation of the entire population of participants available for a particular study. There is a need to develop insight about the ways in which minorities may be excluded and included in any sample population that is used.

One concern of a recent report into REC highlights that their membership may not be representative of the local population (Neuberger 1992). This can mean a lack of appreciation for the value and beliefs of the population likely to be participants in research studies. Equally it is the responsibility of the researcher to be sensitive to the culture, capabilities and value system of potential participants of their research. This may require the provision of PIS and consent forms in more than one language and, for some research participants, interpreters may be needed.

Exclusion of certain minority groups due to language difficulties may mean bias in the sampling frame for a project. The results of research with restrictive or biased samples will not be applicable to the excluded groups. This effectively eliminates them from well researched studies done to indicate optimal treatment and care procedures.

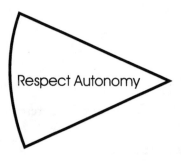

Having respect for the autonomy of people who take part in research means allowing them to determine, of their own free will, whether they will participate in a study. Respecting the autonomy of people is a basic principle of ethical research and is fundamentally linked to the consent procedures the researcher plans to use.

A prime function of informed consent is to support and foster autonomous behaviour. Consent procedures should be worded so that each participant willing agrees to being involved in, and remaining in, the study; and clearly knows what they are agreeing to. This topic is discussed more fully in chapter seven together with the design of PIS and consent forms.

Aspects of consent are also a feature of the duties of the researcher. These are discussed in the following chapter along with a review of the practicalities and outcomes that need consideration in ethically based research. The overlap of consent issues between principles and duties shows the integrative nature of the REW. Whilst no one quarter addresses every ethical issue, certain issues will appear more than once, emphasising their importance in the decision making process.

4
Further principles of research: duty, outcomes and practicalities

4.1 The duties of the researcher

The second quarter of the REW focuses on **deotonology**. Theories associated with this are described as duty ethics. They hold that:

> '*the rightness or wrongness of an act depends neither upon the motive from which the act was done, nor upon the consequences of the act – but solely upon what kind of act it was,*' (Popkin & Stroll 1986, p.56).

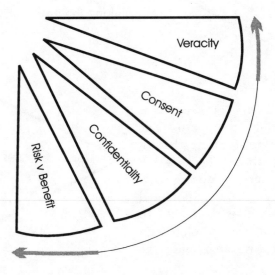

Figure 4.1 The duties of the researcher

The four segments in this quarter, shown in Figure 4.1, are concerned with the duty of the professional towards the people who are asked to consent to participate in research. There is the:

- *Duty of veracity*
- *Duty to carry out research only on those people who have given their valid consent in the presence of a witness*
- *Duty to preserve the anonymity and confidentiality of research participants*
- *Duty, for each participant, to assess the risks against the benefits to be gained.*

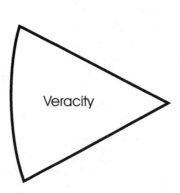

The first two segments in this quarter are very linked with the issue of obtaining consent. This also comes into the segment of the Wheel concerned with respecting the autonomy of people. The overlap highlights how the Wheel encourages more than one way of thinking about research ethics.

The duty of veracity is about telling the truth. The researcher must ensure that all the facts about the research proposal are known and understood by potential participants. It is their duty to ensure that the whole truth about the research and the

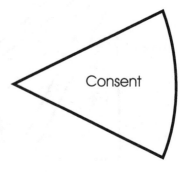

potential effects of any interventions are available. The whole truth means:

- *Clearly stating all the facts*
- *Omitting no information even though you may think it unimportant*
- *Taking care not to use misleading words or phrases.*

The provision of an acceptable PIS and timely discussion with anyone who has queries about their role in the study are important aspects of telling the truth. A sample PIS is discussed in chapter seven where informed consent is more fully debated using examples from PIS that have been offered for use in past studies.

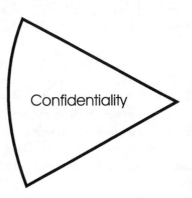
Confidentiality

The third segment in the **duty** quarter is concerned with confidentiality and anonymity. It is the duty of the practitioner undertaking research to ensure that all details relating to the participants in a study remain confidential, and anonymity of participants is maintained.

Health and social care practitioners meet the need to keep information about their patients confidential in routine clinical practice. In certain circumstances, in multi-disciplinary team work for example, confidentiality extends to members of the team. Sharing of information given by the patient to individual practitioners ensures that the best possible care is given. Here it is in the patient's best interest that the complete health care team are fully informed for joint decision making.

In teaching situations information must also be shared with those not directly concerned with the individual patient. This may be a local sharing with students on clinical placements who are required to use patients or their case-notes for learning and assessment purposes. More widely, the submission of anonymous case studies to scientific journals and the display of patient data such as radiographic images during the presentation of posters and papers at conferences is accepted as a way of sharing knowledge within the general health care community.

The use of routine patient data as described above is most usually accepted by patients as either necessary for their immediate care, or helpful in the care of other people in the future. Most understand the need for information to be passed from the ward nurse to the hospital doctor or from the general practitioner to the community physiotherapist. In teaching situations patients have a choice about whether students are present during consultations and care procedures. Students doing assessments must gain the permission of individual patients and few people object to participating in the education of health care professionals in this way.

For those participating in research there is a need for extra consideration about how information gained during the study will be used in their routine care. Patients should know that their general practitioner or hospital consultant will be told if information is found in the study that could influence their future care. They have the right to know that all the information collected about them will be kept confidential, and to whom that confidentiality will extend.

It is important that participants understand that coding on questionnaires and **self-reporting diary cards** results in the collection of information that is not specifically related to them and will not be used to influence their care. Equally important is the need to manage in a sensitive manner, data collected about the staff, and the policies and practices, within an organisation. The researcher must ask how confidential the data they collect will remain by considering:

- *Who else will have access to test results?*
- *Will my supervisor see questionnaire replies?*

- *How identifiable, by a typist, is the data
  collected during interview and sent for
  transcription?*

Where there are few participants in a study, or the work is done within one organisation, it is often possible to recognise people and places. Characteristics of the participants, used in the study as variables or criteria for entry, can lead to identification of who has taken part and/or to the site of the research. The researcher's duty is to highlight these possibilities when gaining consent from potential participants and when asking permission to proceed from organisational managers. The participants should know that whilst they will not be identified by name they may be recognised, once the work is reported, by deduction.

In most instances, as long as individual people or places are not specifically identified, there will not be a problem. Occasionally, people may feel vulnerable if their views are revealed within a work setting and organisations may not wish to have their policies and practices exposed to a wide audience. It is the duty of all researchers to respect this and, working within ethical principles, to ensure that investigations proceed without compromising individuals or hiding out-of-date and inferior practices. Here is another moral dilemma for the researcher to face where there is no solution or a right or wrong answer. It is a matter of making a judgement about the best possible course of action in a given situation.

Data storage methods and reporting mechanisms, including the publication and presentation of papers, must ensure complete anonymity to individual participants. This may require:

- *Developing a coding system for any papers that
  could be attributed to individual participants
  e.g. returned questionnaires, completed data
  sheets on* **performance status**
- *Limiting access of research data to only those
  who are involved with the research and who
  understand the confidential nature of the data*

they are handling, this could include secretaries, statisticians and other staff who help with coding data collected in field studies

- *Recognising the need for security after completion of the study by giving thought to where the information is stored and whether it is appropriate to destroy primary data once the study is complete* (Royal College of Physicians 1990, [i])

- *Respecting the privacy of research participants when the work is submitted for publication by checking for proper names and titles of people and places.*

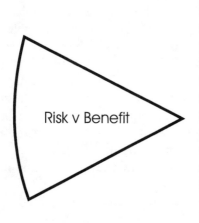

The last segment in this quarter is concerned with the researcher's duty to ensure the protection of research subjects from unnecessary investigation which cannot benefit them or anyone else. It also involves making sure that any risks associated with the proposed study have been minimised to only those necessary to achieve the research objective.

A thorough risk versus benefit analysis on the effect of the research on the participant should be done before the project commences. In doing this the researcher is applying the principle of **beneficence** which includes not inflicting evil or harm. Another way of looking at this is to view the right thing to do as that which will produce the greatest amount of good.

The Declaration of Helsinki (1.5) reminds us that the interests of the subject must take precedence over the interests of society. This is an ideal concept on which to base judgements about who will benefit and who may face a risk from research. It is also helpful to distinguish between the different aims of research studies, and in particular, the difference between studies that aim to:

> *Discover whether a particular intervention is useful*
> *for a given group of people and in doing so will use*
> *that intervention for the potential benefit of some of*
> *those people; a controlled clinical trial of a new drug*
> *versus conventional treatment would come into this*
> *group*

and those that aim to:

> *Discover the effectiveness of a given approach to*
> *routine patient care without altering the intervention;*
> *a patient administered diary about pain and*
> *well-being following cardiac surgery would come into*
> *this group.*

The risk benefit analyses for the two contrasting investigations given above require different approaches. In the first study there is a potential risk that the new drug may not be as effective as the conventional treatment **and** that it could produce unwelcome side-effects in those patients who receive it. These risks must be weighed against the possible advantages of the new drug to the group who receive it, and the potential benefit to future patients.

Advances in the care and management of patients are only possible if risks are taken, if patients are willing, with knowledge of all the facts about a potential new treatment, to participate in research. It is the researcher's duty to assess the risks and the possible benefits and to honestly explain these to potential participants.

In the second study the risk to the patient who participates is likely to be minimal but should not be discounted. Completing diary cards can be stressful and may produce anxiety about **not doing it right, not understanding certain questions and making a mistake.** Some patients may think that what they write will be used **against them** and many fail to realise that the data is being collected generally and not to assist with their particular post-operative care. In this example the benefit of collecting such information is only to future patients but the risk to those participating is small. This type of work is a valid way of advancing the practice of health care and the researcher, again, is asked to make a moral judgement about risk to the individual against potential benefit to the many other patients who may have cardiac surgery.

Finally, in this section, it is worthwhile to consider a group of studies, similar to the second example used above, which may be carried out under the title of *clinical audit*. This type of investigative work has increased considerably since the introduction of the internal health market. It usually involves surveys and questionnaires, with, for example, patients asked to report on their care in particular and the health care environment in general. Whether or not such studies require ethical scrutiny is a local decision often based on the false premise that completing a questionnaire or being interviewed is harmless.

One danger in this approach, for the participants and the researcher, is that the instruments used to gather such data are not scrutinised sufficiently. This can result in data collection tools that fail to meet **reliability** and **validity** criteria and a study which does not conform to accepted scientific method(s). You should be wary of proceeding with studies that are permitted under the audit umbrella and thus escape scientific and ethical scrutiny by an experienced group of people. The appraisal of research by a REC is beneficial to the research process. It is not a confrontational process but one aimed to assist with ensuring that a study is sound and worthwhile.

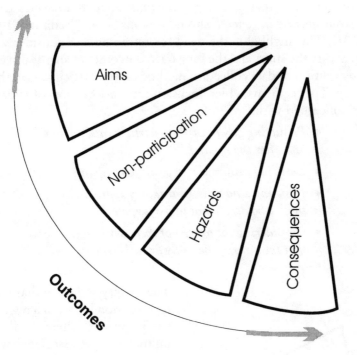

Figure 4.2 The outcome of research

4.2 Outcomes of research

The third quarter of the REW, shown in Figure 4.2, focuses on the consequences of the study that is planned. The theory about consequences and ethical principles holds that:

> 'the rightness or wrongness of an action depends
> entirely upon the effects which the action has,'
> (Popkin & Stroll 1986, p.55).

Ethicists stress that '*not merely the immediate consequences ... but the consequences in general*' should be considered (Seedhouse 1988, p.137). This highlights the need for researchers to consider with equal care the short and the long term outcomes of any health care intervention or data collection method on the participants in their study. The segments which focus on the consequences of research are concerned with:

- *Predicting any hazards to participants, during and after the research*
- *Ensuring minimal risk to all participants*
- *Ensuring a non-discriminatory approach to those who decide not to participate*
- *Considering the process of their work to ensure that the aims of the study are achievable.*

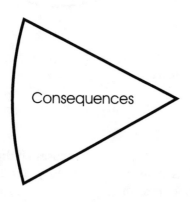

The very fact that an intervention is part of a research study means there will be unknown facts associated with it, linked to the risks of research previously discussed.

The researcher needs to be satisfied that the hazards involved are believed to be predictable. They should stop the investigation if the '*hazards are found to outweigh the potential benefits,*' (Declaration of Helsinki, 1.7.).

Participants in the study have a right to know that there may be hazards and measures must be in place to highlight negative outcomes.

This is where the local REC has an important role. They are directed to consider, '*Are there possible hazards and, if so, adequate facilities to deal with them,*' (Department of Health 1991, p.11). The

PIS must honestly cover matters relating to the risks of research studies. This aspect was previously discussed in relation to the duty to assess risk versus benefit and to ways of ensuring the autonomy of potential research participants. The overlap between different quarters and segments of the Wheel gives you different ways of debating and deciding on how to ensure that your research work is ethically sound.

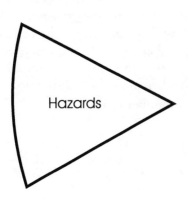

Another segment in the third quarter focuses on the responsibility to ensure that procedures used in health care research do not *'carry a risk which is more than minimal,'* (Royal College of Physicians 1990, [i] p.9). Here the meaning of the word is expanded to include an appreciation of what constitutes minimal risk.

This can be defined as either a negligible risk, i.e. lower than would be met in everyday life, of psychological or physical distress; or a remote probability that serious injury or death will result from participation in the study.

Researchers need to ask themselves questions about the level of invasion and/or intrusion that will be experienced by the participant. Where the risk is significant research cannot be justified since to place participants at such risk violates their autonomy (Beauchamp & Childress 1983).

In the third outcomes segment the researcher is asked to consider the consequences for participants who refuse, for any reason, to participate in their study. The person who decides they cannot take part should not feel that this will lead to discrimination (now or in the future) or that their participation is the only way of receiving optimal treatment.

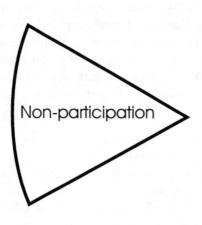

Health and social care professionals will be all too aware that many patients feel they should please the professional, as if this in some way will mean a better outcome of the care offered. The process of consenting people into studies requires that researchers are sensitive to the rather natural wish we all have to be helpful rather than difficult, compliant rather than contrary, especially when in a vulnerable position.

Patients may decline for any number of reasons:

- *Lack of time*
- *Fear of the unknown*
- *Lack of energy for anything other than getting better*
- *A previous poor experience as a research participant.*

In reality, few people refuse and most agree to participate knowing that the results of the study will not directly benefit them. This is well demonstrated by looking at the participation of children with acute lymphatic leukaemia in the national trials that have now been in place many years. Almost all parents, despite the seriousness of the diagnosis and the severity of the interventions, consent to their children entering the studies. Even when their children are in the poor prognosis groups the propensity is to participate and at least help to add to the body of knowledge on the topic.

The Declaration of Helsinki (ii.4) asserts that *'refusal ... to participate ... must never interfere with the physician-patient relationship.'* This applies equally to all care professionals. Delivery of the best health care is dependant upon the integrity of the relationship between patients and their carers. Research into future interventions must not be allowed to damage the effectiveness of present treatments and procedures. A related issue is the consequence for participants who withdraw from a study. They must be assured that they can do so *'at any time without prejudicing their clinical care,'* (Gillet 1990, p.893).

Where studies involve staff or students it is equally important to give people as much choice to participate as not to participate. In health care and educational organisations the hierarchical structure can influence the co-operation of junior staff. Willingness to help a colleague may lead us all into areas we wished we had thought about just a little bit more.

Change is a prevalent feature of today's organisations and questionnaires asking about coping strategies and stress can seem threatening. Some people may fear exposure if they answer your questions honestly. It is worthwhile remembering that the unwilling participant is most likely to be an unreliable informant or respondent: and you may lose a valued colleague if they feel unduly pressured into participating with your research.

It is the duty of the researcher to ensure that participation and withdrawal are voluntary. This includes being sensitive during follow-up enquiries to unreturned questionnaires and remembering to tell potential participants that they can change their mind about being involved at any time. This is why many REC not only scrutinise research proposals with patients as participants but also those that involve health authority staff and students.

Other organisations, such as universities, where staff and students are routinely involved in research are now following the lead of health authorities in this way. If you are a student embarking on a research project it is now more common to find that you will need ethical clearance from your faculty or university before you proceed with an investigation. Of course if your work involves patients from a NHS trust hospital then you are also likely to need ethical clearance from their REC.

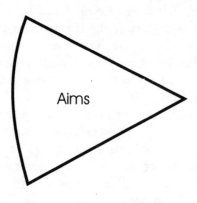

Finally in this quarter there is the reminder that ethical research is that where the aims of the research process are achievable. This is similar to the need to be guided by scientific principles referred to in the first quarter of the REW. Research that fails to produce *'useful or valid results'* is unethical (Denham 1979, p.1043).

Another role of REC is to reject proposals that do not have a *'reasonable chance of answering the question under examination,'* (British Association of Occupational Therapists 1990 [ii] p.5).

4.3 Practicalities of the research process

Figure 4.3 shows the segments in the fourth quarter of the REW. These are directed towards consideration of the external environment and place ethical decision making within the context of limitations and doubt (Seedhouse 1988, 138-9).

Included are:

- *Codes of practice and the law*
- *The need to consider the researcher's ability to carry out the study*
- *The obligation to optimise use of resources*
- *The necessity for independent scrutiny of research proposals and publication of results.*

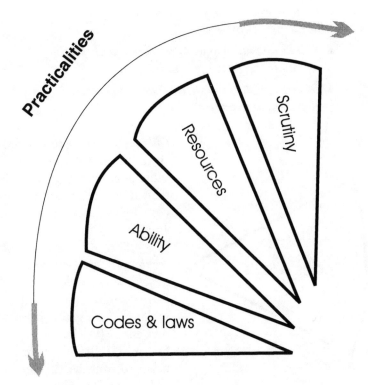

Figure 4.3 The practicalities of the research process

All health care workers, whether participating in routine work or in research, are guided by their professional code of practice. Many health and social care professional organisations issue guidance on research ethics and other information e.g. notes on applying to REC. Graduate entry into the PSMs, and inclusion of graduate qualifications within the education structure of nursing and other care practitioners, has seen a welcome rise in the interest of professional bodies in research based practice. The need for well planned and carefully executed studies into all health and social care practice was fully discussed earlier. Professional organisations have a role in providing:

- *Policies which encourage practitioner and academic research*
- *Guidance and support to enable researchers to negotiate the gatekeepers to research*
- *Rigorous codes of research practice to enhance the status of their researchers.*

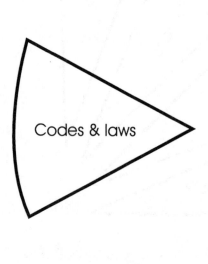

Codes & laws

Of course, provision is only the beginning. It is then up to individual investigators to be guided, to follow advice and contribute the results of their enquiries.

The *'laws and regulations of the country in which the research experiment is performed'* must not be violated during the research process (Declaration of Helsinki, 1.2). The researcher needs to consider the issue of indemnity offered to research participants in relation to the health authority and companies associated with the research. It also means that researchers are obliged to follow the accepted practice of the country in which the study is done with regard to obtaining permission to begin investigative work.

In the United Kingdom the ethical scrutiny of research studies is not governed by law. Health authorities are advised by DOH guidelines which set out ways in which this type of scrutiny should be done. Whilst these are sufficient in many localities, and do ensure that patients and healthy volunteers recruited into research studies are protected, there are differences in how the guidelines are implemented. Problems often arise with the scrutiny of multi-centred studies and health services research; problems that would be diminished if all health authorities were obliged to follow the same set of rules and standards set by a national ethics committee (NEC).

Researchers need to be aware of the local differences in the application of these guidelines and the implications of such individuality for the efficient and effective scrutiny of their studies. In chapters six and seven guidance is given on ways to ensure that your application to REC following the DOH guidelines is successful.

To meet many of the criteria mentioned in previous segments of the REW it is vital that ethical scrutiny includes an assurance *'that the people responsible for the research are well qualified to do it,'* (Neuberger 1992, p. 37).

There are several dimensions to the competency and capability of researchers, these include:

- *Awareness of present knowledge on the topic*

- *Ability to use the appropriate data collection tools for a particular study*

- *Provision of sound research supervision and an understanding by the researcher of the role of the supervisor.*

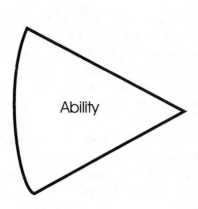

All of this is supported by the suggestion that it is the responsibility of a REC to satisfy itself that the 'project ... (is) within the competence of the research workers concerned,'(Northern Regional Health Authority Working Group 1978). Meaningful investigations are those supported by information on the current state of knowledge on the research topic. Proposals that do not indicate appraisal of the literature and an ability to analyse several, sometimes conflicting sources, will be seen as unsound. The researcher needs to set their work in the context of the work of other investigators, to compliment other studies and to build on prior and preliminary work. Consideration of these aspects will lead to ethically and scientifically sound research.

This segment also highlights the need for research capability by the investigator(s). It is usually clear whether those investigating pure science, often in a laboratory setting, have the necessary technical skills to undertake the processes involved in data collection and experimentation. In such instances students or novice researchers are usually closely supervised to ensure personal health and safety, and the careful use of expensive instrumentation.

In contrast, the design and administration of questionnaires and interviews can be seen as relatively easy. Indeed, many undergraduate students embarking on a project opt for these survey techniques. There is a mistaken belief that anyone can compose a few questions and that interviewing for research purposes is very similar to communicating with people in general. But questionnaire design is a complex task with the mistakes of those who have not studied this method in detail frequently appearing only when the replies are analysed. It is unethical to expect patients or staff to spend time completing a questionnaire that yields very little useful data.

In a similar way, researchers need to be aware of the skills involved in conducting either, structured, semi-structured, or unstructured interviews. In these situations people are frequently asked searching questions, inviting them to think deeply about personal issues. Hancock (1994, p.44) reminds us that this can open up a *'can of worms ... without any follow up or support'*.

Researchers have an ethical responsibility towards their participants during, and following, interview. Some interviewers may not have the time or competence to deal with any problems that arise during the time they spend with research participants. Some may find the boundary between the caring professional and the objective researcher difficult to set. Such issues need consideration before the start of a study if it is to proceed in an ethically sound manner.

National guidelines require REC to ask the question whether the investigation is properly supervised and the supervisor adequately qualified and experienced (Department of Health 1991). For work done towards an academic award the provision of a supervisor is usually the responsibility of course organisers and many new researchers, fortunately, find themselves working alongside more experienced colleagues.

The unfortunate few, often where research into clinical practice is a new and untried concept, may find themselves alone and with little guidance or help. The risk in this situation is that the investigative work will be flawed and the researcher is well advised to find someone, possibly in another organisation, who is willing to provide supervision. Whatever the source of your supervision it is your responsibility to make use of the advice and help that is given; to accept that research is a complex and scientific process with skills and knowledge that need to be learnt.

Research is resource intensive and ethical scrutiny of a study would be incomplete without consideration of the effect it may

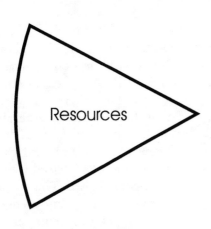

have on associated work. Equally important is the need for accurate and detailed costing of all investigative work. Undergraduate students should consider whether the time and materials are available for them to carry out their chosen study and, if not, who is to meet any expenses for their work.

Currently, all work within the NHS is subject to resource management. This approach should include measuring how productive research work is, by the staff responsible for establishing any study. Review of the capital and revenue consequences of research is vital together with ensuring that all that is needed for successful completion of the study will be available. The process of ethical scrutiny includes a responsibility to ensure that the research will be done within suitable premises and that suitable facilities are available to design the study and to collect and analyse data.

This segment in the fourth quarter of the Wheel, with its focus on resources, overlaps with the principle of working on a sound scientific basis towards improving knowledge and understanding. Considering the practicalities of the research process together with that principle will guard against the researcher not fulfilling their *'obligation in justice not to engage in research which is valueless and is a waste of time and resources,'*(Thompson et al 1988, p.167). Disregarding the principle and the practicalities could invite abuse of resources, especially where funding for research is competitive and researchers also have a routine clinical role.

Finally, the last segment in the fourth quarter emphasises that before any research study commences it is imperative that it is considered by an independent committee in order that, *'Investigators should not be the sole judge of whether their research ...*

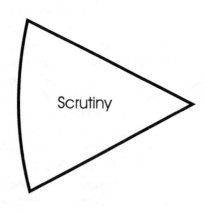

conform(s)' to codes of research practice such as the Declaration of Helsinki (Royal College of Physicians 1990, [ii] p.1). And after completion there is an obligation to publish accurate results and to analyse data in an independent and unbiased way (Declaration of Helsinki and Dickenson 1991). This wide sharing of knowledge, whether positive or negative, is fundamental to the progress of health and social care. Unpublished research may prevent out-of-date procedures being replaced by new and more effective research-based regimes. Work that lies dormant on the bookshelf and is not shared with others may lead to the wasteful repetition of studies.

Failure to publish is detrimental to the progress of recognising new paradigms of research. Individual work that remains unknown to the wider community of academics and practitioners fails to support research based education in health care. Inviting and learning from critical comments by means of wide publication gives coherence to the newer, non-positivistic perspectives on health care.

5
Ethical and scientific scrutiny: who are the gatekeepers?

5.1 Gatekeepers in the research process

At the very beginning of a piece of research, when the idea is just a faint glimmer in your head and before you start to make decisions about how you are going to do the work there are some practical issues that are well worth your time and careful thought. Some important questions to answer at this early stage are:

- *Is what I want to do research?*
- *Who is it going to involve as participants?*
- *Who am I going to have to convince about the value and importance of investigating the topic?*

One common element in research by all health and social care professional workers is the necessary involvement of people or their case notes in some way. Whatever the nature of your enquiry, if it relates to people, then you are responsible for ensuring that the work is ethically and scientifically sound. Some of the ways in which people may be participants within a research project are as:

patients	clients
family of patients or clients	colleagues
students	members of the general public

you are unsure about the nature of the work you are doing ask yourself these questions:

- *What is the intention of this work?*
- *Does the work only involve caring for the patient or is it also evaluation of that care?*
- *Will I acquire the knowledge to change practice by the methods I plan to use to do this work?*
- *Does the work involve some form of investigation into how people think, behave or feel?*

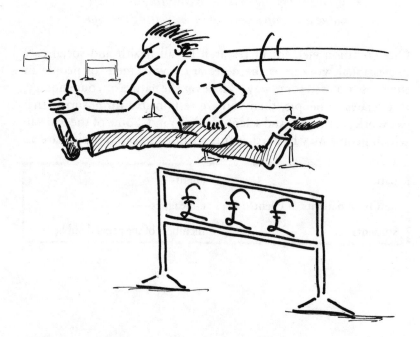

Figure 5.1 Gatekeepers in the research process

Your replies should help you to answer the question, **Am I undertaking research?**

If the answer to this question is **yes, I am** then it is essential that permission to proceed is sought from the relevant authorities. Figure 5.1 shows that whatever you are doing there are likely to be a number of gatekeepers that you need to negotiate with before your research begins. They will vet your proposal before you involve people as participants in your investigation and start the data collection.

You should not see gatekeeping as the process of putting hurdles in your way or placing a trip wire in your path to publication. Neither does the process of vetting research proposals aim to prevent you from finding the answers to the questions you're asking about your professional practice. Each gatekeeper is likely to help you in some way and you should take advantage of this. At the same time they will also highlight for you some of the difficulties and dilemmas presented by your initial ideas about your study. Do use their expertise and experience. Be grateful that someone has pointed out to you, sooner rather than later, that one of your ideas won't work or that this study has already been done. Most research benefits from collaboration and the time spent planning a project is never wasted. A great deal can be gained by **running your ideas** past colleagues and friends who are willing to play **devils advocate** with your previously well thought out study design (Figure 5.2)!

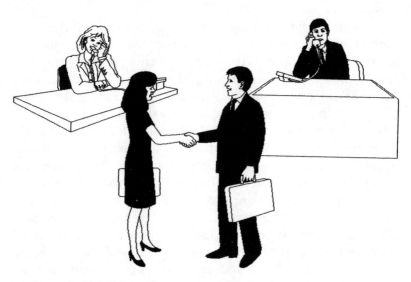

Figure 5.2 Talking about your ideas

The gatekeepers to your research may include:

- *Your personal tutor, course director and academic board of studies if you are studying for a diploma or degree*

- *Your line manager and/or head of department with responsibility for use of resources (time and money) in your place of work, medical colleagues with direct responsibility for patients who are potential participants of your research*

- *Colleagues in health and social care who collaborate in the care of potential participants of your research*
- *Official committees within your institution or health authority with responsibility for the ethical and scientific scrutiny of research.*

As the list shows the roles and responsibilities of all these potential gatekeepers are varied. There are formal groups of people who may not be known to you at all and individual people with whom you may already have a good working and friendly relationship. Earlier research work may have given you the experience of discussing a project with some of them. This may be the first time you have had to initiate meetings with the direct intention of asking permission or co-operation to proceed with research.

Before you start to talk to anyone think ahead about the best approach for each of the different gatekeepers. Remember that you should have a clear idea about what you want to do by this time: an idea or ideas that are flexible and ready to be shaped by guidance from colleagues and academic staff but which indicate that you have already given time and thought to your planned project. At the very least you should know:

- *The questions you want your research to answer*
- *Why you want to know those answers.*

With close colleagues it is always helpful to have an early and informal chat about what you are doing. Offer to follow this up with an outline of your research plans. Some people like to have something in writing to record their discussion with you. Others may be happy to chat again when necessary and might file your outline project proposal in the waste paper bin! Whatever they want, it is always worth keeping a short record of your discussions with these more informal gatekeepers. In this way you know who has offered what advice and help for the future.

5.2 Formal and official gatekeepers

Having outlined some of the less formal barriers to your research work this chapter now looks at the structures set up to formally scrutinise research proposals.

Gatekeepers who need to give their express permission before any research begins within your institution need to be approached more formally. The clinician or manager responsible for any patients or people who may be participants in your project is likely to want a written outline of your aims and objectives, and some information about the design of the study. Anyone asked to provide resources for a project will want a statement of why the funds are needed and how any money allocated for your research will be spent.

This applies whether you are asking a university department for a small amount of money to cover the cost of paper and postage for questionnaires or an external funding organisation for money to meet the salary costs of a data processing clerk. Academic boards, REC and scientific review committees (SRC) usually have forms for researchers to complete and many require extra information, such as the consent form, to be attached.

The REC and the SRC are likely to be less familiar to novice researchers than their colleagues or manager are. These committees are formal bodies accountable to the highest authorities within institutions and can be rather awesome to approach. Chapters six and seven give more detailed information on the process of obtaining ethical clearance. Doing something for the first time, especially when it involves senior colleagues in official positions can be daunting. The more you know about the background to the processes and people involved the better you will be able to prepare yourself and any documents.

The remainder of this chapter looks at the history of research ethics and the development of the process of reviewing the ethics of research. It concludes with details about the committees that scrutinise research to ensure that it is ethically sound. With knowledge of who sits on these committees and how they work the task of making an application will be easier.

5.3 Research ethics committees: history and pre structure

In the United Kingdom permission to proceed wi research should be sought from your local REC. These committees are charged with advising on '*all matters pertaining to the ethics of research involving human subjects,*'(Royal College of Physicians 1990, [ii]p.7). Their function is to guarantee that all health related research is appraised and monitored so that high ethical standards are maintained. Their remit includes all health care research relating to persons including the use of questionnaires and existing records. Not only do they grant approval but may, if necessary, withdraw it.

The function of the REC extends beyond simple approval to include:

- *Ensuring that the participant freely volunteers to take part in research projects*
- *Protecting those who refused to participate*
- *Safeguarding the autonomy of participants*
- *Resource issues*
- *Mechanisms for ongoing appraisal of research studies.*

The process of ethical scrutiny by committee is relatively recent. Many were established in the late 1960's after a suggestion by the Ministry of Health for peer review of research projects and some unspecific guidance on how this might be done from the Royal College of Physicians. Advice and reports on granting ethical clearance to researchers who use patients or patient related data in their studies have been regular features of state and professional bodies since then. One thing that REC appear to have in common is that one is not likely to be like another. If you have applied to a REC in one health district and are now working elsewhere your past experience may be different from the one you are about to have. Nevertheless, your previous experience will still be helpful.

Surveys of REC in 1981, 1988 and 1989 indicated diversity in their practice and this remains a feature of the most recent report (Neuberger 1992). A study of Scottish REC revealed a *'considerable and confusing lack of uniformity in arrangements for the different types of ethical committees,'* (Thompson et al 1981, p.719).

There are also differences in the operation of the REC surveyed in Scotland to that of a REC in an English health authority (Denham et al 1979). A sample of 28 REC in England showed a diversity in many characteristics including size of committee and ethical criteria, guidance given to research workers and in the information asked of them (Gilbert et al 1989). The authors were also concerned that *'guidelines ... have been widely ignored,'* (Gilbert et al 1989 p.1438). The frequency of meetings may vary considerably and the REC may not meet the guidelines about lay membership (Nott & Steel 1988).

All these differences mean that applicants for ethical clearance need to find out how their local REC works if they are to put together a successful application. The very best help you can give yourself as a researcher is to find out the **who, when, where and how** of the way the REC in your health district operates.

More generally the differences in REC gives rise to concern about the ability of some health authorities to ensure informed ethical scrutiny for research involving people. Certain types of research studies are seen as problem areas. These include large-scale, multi-centre epidemiological studies and health services projects (Gilbert-Foster 1991).

These so-called problem studies would be less problematic if the very real problem of the *'diversity, and inadequacy in some cases, of ethics committees in this country'* was tackled and solved (Gilbert-Foster 1991, p.230). But if you are involved in the type of research that causes problems, and need REC permission to proceed then, until the present system is changed, you need to know what that is and how to maximise your chances of a successful application.

If you are asked to join a REC then it may be helpful to know where its strengths and weaknesses are likely to be. Your experience may be needed to compliment the present members.

Once an established member you may need to suggest that the committee widens its membership to overcome difficulties with particular types of research.

There is support for the establishment of *'a national committee with policing powers'; 'a national ethics committee (NEC),'* (Gilbert-Foster 1991, p.230; and Warnock 1988, p.1626). This national body would *'be concerned with a … range of ethical problems, arising in both medical practice and research,'* (Warnock 1988, p.1626).

It has been suggested, that for multi-centre studies, the local REC would still have the right not to give permission for projects approved by a NEC if they were unconvinced about their ethical soundness. In addition, the establishment of a NEC could provide a system for regulating REC, and sanctioning those who *'fail to keep to agreed standards,'* (Lock 1990).

In addition to a policing role an NEC could provide a *'forum for debate and discussion' 'information and advice'* and a way of enabling the *'experience and expertise of the established REC to be shared,'* (Gilbert Foster 1992, p.11).

It may well be that the law will soon replace advice and there are good reasons for this happening in the 1990's. There is increasing public interest in health matters, particularly in relation to control and choice. The introduction of the Patients Charter means that the Government is willing to be active in supporting patients rights in health care. This will surely include the fundamental right to informed and consensus ethical scrutiny of research involving patients. This may lead to the legal requirement for ethical review and approval as practised in the United States of America (Levine 1989).

Another difference in the operational nature of REC is whether they work separately from a committee for scientific review. This is another item on your check list of what you need to find out about the local process of ethical scrutiny.

A SRC exists to assess the scientific aspects of a research proposal. The members of this committee look at features of the research proposal such as:

- *The study design*
- *Methods of data collection*
- *Reliability and validity*
- *The contribution of the proposed work to the present body of knowledge on the topic of the research.*

With thorough assessment of the scientific aspects of each proposal already complete the ethics committee can concentrate on aspects of proposals that relate more closely to those who will participate in the research. With the rigor and scientific soundness already examined there is time at ethics committees for closer scrutiny of the moral and participant related consequences of the research. The split of scientific and ethical scrutiny allows the latter rightly to be the focus of the ethics committee.

The responsibility for establishing a REC rests with the District Health Authority (DHA) in consultation with other health care organisations within its boundaries. The REC is then responsible for the ethical scrutiny of all research involving patients within that area. This responsibility is irrespective of where the study is done and who does the work; it is related to the participants of the research and the geographical focus of their care. Some studies, especially those that investigate rare or unusual diseases with a low incidence, often need to recruit participants from many health authorities. These multi-centre projects, organised from one institution, need to apply to individual REC for permission to proceed with the patients registered in their particular authority. Other features of REC include:

- *Accountability to the DHA*
- *Making an annual report available to the public and the press*
- *Membership of 8-12*
- *Equal representation from both sexes and all ages*

- *The need for the membership to reflect the local population*
- *Representation across all health care disciplines*
- *Lay members or member of the public who are not health professionals.*

Some REC meet the guidelines recommended for membership and have all of the features listed above. With others it is likely that the membership is not *'representative of the multi-professional research which it has become their task to adjudge,'* (Schröck 1991, p38). A balanced and informed REC needs to have amongst its members those who can scrutinise a wide range of research designs that use the spectrum of methodologies available in the natural and social sciences. In particular health services researchers would particularly like to see *'statisticians, social scientists, epidemiologists and managers'* included in the membership of a REC (Ginzler et al 1990, p.195).

The members of the REC are there to:

- *Assess research proposals in a constructive manner*
- *Have a regard for the truth*
- *Be aware and sensitive to the different values of all potential research participants.*

You may know some of the members of your local REC through your work. It is less likely that you will have met the lay members who are appointed to the Committee to:

- *Balance the needs of medical research and potential participants of investigative work*
- *Give a non-medical view of the proposed research*
- *Ensure that PIS and consent forms are free from professional jargon and will be understood by the research participants.*

In the past the hospital chaplain often took the role of lay member. Although such persons can provide an ethical viewpoint it is better if lay people are not employees of the health authority. It is now more common for lay members to be well informed members of the public with an interest in health care and ethics. The health authority might appoint a member of the Community Health Council to the REC or a lawyer with a medico-legal interest. Sometimes the chairperson of the Committee is a lay member and this can be seen as a very sound way of protecting the interests of research participants.

This chapter has highlighted the barriers that need to be negotiated at the beginning of a research project. Your role in the research community, the topic and potential participants of your study, will all influence which individuals and groups need to give you permission to proceed with your research. All of this can take considerable time and can be quite stressful. Good planning is essential, especially if your work has to be completed within the time set by an award course. The next chapter tells you more about the formal process of obtaining scientific and ethical clearance and how to help yourself make this as smooth as possible.

6
Applying for ethical clearance

This chapter aims to help you make a successful application for ethical clearance and gain permission to go ahead with your research. In the previous chapter the different ways health authorities establish committees for this purpose was described. It is important to find out about the local arrangements for ethical scrutiny since these will affect the way your application is processed.

You may be applying to one committee, a REC, or to two committees, a REC and a SRC so knowing what happens in the local health authority is important. Help with making an application is almost always available, as indicated in later sections of this chapter. The best means of making the most of the expertise and experience your colleagues may offer is also looked at. Your application is more likely to succeed if you scrutinise your proposal first, guided by some knowledge of ethical principles and a check list of issues likely to be considered by the REC. All these ways which contribute towards a successful application are discussed below.

6.1 Information on local arrangements

First of all, check that there is either a REC or both an REC and SRC within the health authority you work for, with responsibility for people who may be participants of your research. In the unlikely event of not finding one, students doing research as part of an award course should look to see if their University or College has an ethics committee. It is becoming more common for universities and other higher education institutions to establish committees for the purpose of ethical scrutiny.

Ghazi and Cook (1993, p.27) describe the setting up of a Research, Ethics and Consultative Committee in a College of Health Studies which as well as providing *'guidance and support to staff and students wanting to undertake research'* also monitors research activity *'particularly in relation to ethical considerations'*. You may be required to put your proposal to the education REC before proceeding onto the health authority REC. If so, do ask if the education REC will accept the application form used by the health authority REC.

It is wise to begin the process of getting ethical clearance as soon as you can. It may take some time for your application to circulate to the members of an REC which operates by post only. Of REC who hold meetings, some do so infrequently e.g. four times a year and some take a long summer break. All of this could delay the start of your study.

Most Committees have a secretary, usually someone working for the health authority who will give you details of how to apply. The secretary will also advise on whether there are local regulations which permit particular studies to be passed by *chair's action* alone. If you can't find the name of the secretary try to contact the chairperson or one of the other committee members. It is unlikely that anyone will refuse to give you details of how the committee operates though the secretary will probably be your best source of information. At this stage you will find it helpful to know:

- *The dates of REC and/or SRC meetings*
- *The time before the REC meeting by which applications must be submitted*
- *The application procedure.*

Of the committees that hold meetings, there are some where the written applications only are discussed, and in exceptional circumstances researchers interviewed. Others invite all researchers for interview to discuss the application. Make sure you know how often applications are looked at and the average time it takes to process one. With this information you can plan the process of applying to ensure that the start of your project is not delayed.

During the process of getting ethical clearance there are several stages at which you may find some advice helpful. These include:

- *Completing the application form*
- *Writing any additional papers required by the REC, such as a PIS*
- *Preparing for an interview.*

Colleagues who have made successful applications will probably be willing to discuss their experiences with you and REC members may be willing to help. The expertise and experience of the members is very valuable and most see helping novice applicants as part of their role.

6.2 The application form

Novice researchers may find completing an application form for ethical clearance rather daunting. The process can be easier if you:

- *Make some copies to complete in draft. It often takes more than one attempt to put all the information about your study onto the form provided. Being prepared for this can help to reduce the stress (Figure 6.1)*
- *Enquire whether the form is available on computer disk. This allows flexibility of fitting your proposal into space allocated for different sections on the form and reduces typographical wear and tear*
- *Read the accompanying instructions carefully. Some committees ask you to send them multiple copies and others will ask for the information to be typed or written in black ink for clear*

copying and make their own copies for
distribution to all REC members

- Remember that the form was probably designed
  for clinical/quantitative studies. This can
  present difficulties with some sections if you are
  using a different type of research methodology.
  You need to use your **common-sense** and may
  have to **interpret** the form with some flexibility!

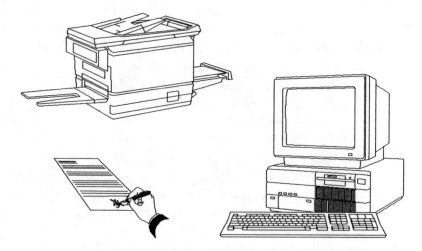

Figure 6.1 Practice makes perfect!

If you have difficulty understanding what is required in each section try to find out what other researchers did. It is especially helpful to discuss your application with someone who has used the same methodological approach to data collection and analysis that you plan to use.Complete the form as accurately and fully as possible. Some committees require all the questions to be answered; it is insufficient to refer them to your protocol. Take note of any papers associated with your study that the Committee expects to be appended to the application form. An incomplete application may be delayed. Submission of insufficient information about the proposed study can mean postponement to a later meeting of the REC. The committee are likely to want to see:

- *The study protocol or proposal*
- *The PIS*
- *A non-standard consent form*
- *Draft questionnaires and semi-structured interview questions*
- *A signed statement from any commercial company supplying a drug which does not have Product Liability Insurance (PLI) saying that it abides by the 1993 guidelines of the Association of the British Pharmaceutical Industry (ABPI) of the APBIs's code of practice.*

Tasks such as completing the application form can be very time consuming and it is vital to keep the deadline date for submission in mind. In some instances you may need to have sections of the form, or separate statements, signed by a number of different people, including:

- *Your manager with evidence of support for time and other resources*
- *Clinical consultant(s) with responsibility for patients who may be participants in your study*

- *Heads of departments that have agreed to any
  extra cost/work as the result of involvement
  with your study*
- *Your research supervisor.*

All this can take extra time and failing to catch the right person just before they take a few days annual leave may mean a delay in starting your study.

What to do if there is no application form

Without an application form you are left to decide for yourself what the REC might wish to know about the study you plan to do. Include as much detail as possible but be aware of the need to keep your application concise. It will be read by busy people who may suffer quickly from information overload, to the detriment of your application!

Most of what you write about your study will include terminology related to the content and process of the research you wish to do. Without this, it is difficult to convey your knowledge and skills to carry out the investigative work. It can be helpful for your application to include a summary of your study written in a way that everyone can understand it, free from professional jargon. This will be appreciated by the lay members and is a good way of demonstrating how you will explain the research to potential participants during the process of getting their informed consent.

6.3 Interviews

If your local committee regularly interviews applicants, find out who is expected to attend since arrangements do vary. Some committees require the medical practitioner responsible for the participants of the study to attend even when they are not the principal investigator. Other committees only see principal investigators. Others having designated staff who may attend and who can accompany junior staff.

A recent study of one REC by Hammick (1993, p.99) revealed a sensitive approach to interviewees by the members, especially to novice researchers who might be *'like frightened rabbits'* (Figure 6.2). REC members in that study spoke of being patient and facilitative and of their role as one of assisting researchers in their work rather than as a block to investigative studies on a broad range of topics.

The interviewing process is seen as a way of assessing the attitude of researchers to investigative work with patients and of actively involving REC members and applicants in the debate about ethical issues. In the work done by Hammick (1993, pp.89-90) REC members thought that member's *'views were modified by the opportunity to discuss the research directly with the investigator'*. Similarly, since interviews had become compulsory for applications to the particular REC investigated by Hammick (1993) much more thought and care had been put into PIS. All this indicates the value of being able to support your application in person.

Yes, attending any interview is daunting, especially for the first time and when your important study depends on the outcome. But being present to support your research design, and having the opportunity to show how you are willing to learn from the expert and experienced comments of the REC, can have very positive benefits for your research.

Interviews give REC members the opportunity to get direct answers to their queries from the researchers often leading to an immediate decision about the application. This saves time not only for the Committee with usually more than enough work to do, but also for the investigators for whom time is often a critical factor in the research process.

It is likely that you will be asked to give a brief (two minute) overview about your research and this will be followed by questions to you from the members. This is your opportunity to demonstrate motivation and commitment to the work. The summary should include why you are doing the study, how you plan to do it and what you expect to find. Some applicants can be too 'technical' or even too 'flippant' in what they say (Hammick 1993, p.99).

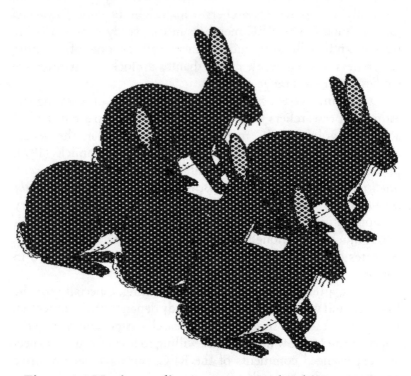

Figure 6.2 Novice applicants to a research ethics committee

Aim for a succinct outline appropriate to the understanding of all
the Committee, including the lay members.

The questions may be on any area of your proposed work;
even if your study has been looked at by an SRC the REC may
still question you about the scientific principles. It is unlikely that
an SRC would ask about ethical issues.

The following list gives some examples of the topics that are raised:

1. Incompatibility of the aims of the study with the planned measures of outcome.

2. Amount of bias in a study when participants know their conversation is being recorded.

3. Prediction of how many patients will refuse to participate in a study.

4. Method of recruiting patients into a study.

5. What will happen to those patients who decide not to participate?

6. How sick are the potential participants of the study?

7. Will the general practitioner be informed about their patients participation?

If you are required to attend for interview, do take a copy of your application with you. You will find this helpful during any reference to it by the REC members and you can note, close to the relevant section, their comments for future use.

If you are to be interviewed try to talk to someone who has local experience of this. They will be able to outline what happens and a little knowledge about what type of questions your REC may ask will help you to feel more at ease.

6.4 Ethical principles for self-scrutiny

As indicated earlier you can carry out your own ethical appraisal of your application to a REC both as self-scrutiny of the documents you submit and mental practice on the questions you might be asked at an interview. In previous chapters the principles behind ethically sound research were examined in detail. The following brief list is written as a guide to some of the issues the REC are likely to raise about your application and how you can help to make your application successful.

First: when you complete the application form or make revisions and during your interview by the REC members it helps if you:

- *give an honest summary of your study*
- *demonstrate attention to the basic principles of research ethics*

Secondly: remember that the REC is likely to focus on three aspects of your study:

- *its impact on the participants (this will probably receive most attention)*
- *content and design of the research proposal*

- *external influences on the work you plan to do*

And: there is a lot of evidence that the REC frequently directs its attention to:

- *ensuring that participants are empowered to give informed consent*
- *protecting participants who wish to withdraw from any study at any time*

- *the clarity of the PIS*

Finally: refer back to chapters three and four for the details of the segments of each quarter of the REW and debate whether the principles, duties, outcomes and practicalities of your study are compatible with ethical research.

The following list reminds you about these:

1. The principles behind research using patients:
   - *A sound scientific basis*
   - *Improvement of knowledge and understanding*
   - *Respecting all persons equally*
   - *Respecting the autonomy of all persons.*

2. The duties of a researcher:
   - *Of veracity or truthfulness*
   - *To carry out research only on those people who have given their valid consent*
   - *To preserve the anonymity and confidentiality of research participants*
   - *To assess the risks against the benefits to be gained.*

3. The nature of the outcome of the research:
   - *Short and long term consequences of the study intervention*
   - *Hazards associated with the research*
   - *Non-discrimination towards those who decide not to participate*
   - *Achievable aims for the study.*

4. The practicalities of the research process:
   - *Following codes of professional practice and the law*
   - *The researchers ability to carry out the study*
   - *Optimising the use of resources*
   - *Ensuring the work is subject to independent scrutiny, and publishing results.*

6.5 Following up the application

REC members, individually and collectively, are there to advise and scrutinise; investigators are responsible for integrating suggestions and advice into their work. There is strong evidence that the principle concern of REC is that potential participants be protected at all cost. They also recognise that they have a duty to encourage research into health care practice.

Listen to their advice and ask for their guidance; there is always more than one way of looking at an issue. The objective view from the other side is usually helpful if we can overcome our instinct to be defensive about a research proposal that has taken many hours to prepare!

If you are required to resubmit your application be positive about the suggestions made by the members and accept their wisdom. Remember to keep a diary of the process of obtaining ethical clearance. You will need to write about this in your final report in the section on gaining access to the participants and permission for your study to take place. Investigators, and participants in research, will benefit from ethical scrutiny by an REC; good luck as you make your way through that process.

This chapter has highlighted ways towards a successful application for ethical clearance which is an essential part of the research process for a study involving people. It is a task that can be stressful even for experienced researchers and daunting for those who are new to the process. The focus on informed consent and the PIS at REC meetings has been mentioned more than once. The next chapter looks at this important part of research using people.

7
Informed consent or telling it exactly how it will be

7.1 Informed consent and research participants

A prime responsibility of every researcher is:

1. Preparation of appropriate papers for the process of obtaining informed consent from people who agree to participate in their study.

2. The sensitive use of these during initial discussions with potential participants about the study and the expected role of the participant in the study.

This chapter looks at several issues surrounding informed consent including the part played by REC and the preparation of straightforward and honest PIS. The format of consent forms is not discussed since, in most settings, research studies involving patients use standard hospital consent forms. Indeed, if you do not plan to use the standard form in use in the organisation in which you work the REC will probably want to know why. Should you find yourself without access to a standard form then it is best to look carefully at one or two of these and formulate your own using the standard forms as a model. It is not advisable to include information for potential participants to your study on a consent form. The PIS should be separate from the consent form.

7.2 Informed consent and research ethics committees

Informed consent is the subject of much discussion by REC. The wording of consent forms, and the documentation prepared to form potential participants about the study, indicates the attitude of the researcher towards informed consent. This, in turn, is linked to their approach to ensuring that the autonomy of the research participants is retained.

A case study of one REC strongly indicated that protecting the autonomy of potential participants was considered to be a major function of the Committee (Hammick 1993). The REC members saw themselves as accountable for:

- *Ensuring that patients made independent decisions with regard to entering studies*
- *Safeguarding the research participants autonomy throughout their participation in a project.*

Other literature on the process of ethical scrutiny gives examples of the attention given to informed consent. For example:

- *'The main concerns REC members referred to as "ethical" (sic) were largely related to consent,' (Neuberger 1992, p. 43)*
- *A review of REC in Scotland found that 20 of the 28 committees who took part in the survey encountered ethical problems related to consent* (Thompson et al 1981)
- *A survey of 28 of the 190 REC in England, found that informed consent was 'the only criterion mentioned by all the committees that provided information' to applicants in a printed format* (Gilbert et al 1989, p.1438).

It is an essential task of an REC *'to decide whether and how the subjects of research will be able to give free informed consent,'* (College of Psychiatrists 1990, p.48). Many studies are supported by the pharmaceutical industry. They also recommend that REC consider that 'appropriate informed consent will be obtained,' (ABPI 1990, p.4).

Guidelines on research ethics by public, professional and commercial organisations devote a lot of space to consent issues.

Two reports from the Royal College of Physicians each devote a chapter to the topic. One stresses the status of the patient by stating that:

> *'Patients should be invited to participate in research as volunteers in the same way as healthy individuals are invited to volunteer,'* (Royal College of Physicians 1990, [i] p.15).

The other highlights the protective functions of written consent:

> *'for subjects (who are in no doubt they are entering research), and for investigators (where evidence of written consent may render them less vulnerable to litigation),'* (Royal College of Physicians 1990, [ii] p.20).

This section has shown the importance of informed consent from the viewpoint of professional bodies and the committees responsible for scrutinising and monitoring research studies. The next section looks in detail at informed consent as a concept in itself. The aim is to help with the understanding of some of the complex issues that surround informed consent. It can seem a simple procedure but without attention to detail some of the fundamental rights of potential research participants can be breached.

7.3 The concept of informed consent

The concept of informed consent is complex and controversial. Its complexity is well demonstrated by the need to see it as having two elements:

- *Informational elements of disclosure and comprehension*

- *Consent elements of voluntariness and competence* (Beauchamp & Childress 1983).

The controversy is associated with ensuring that *'consent (is) freely given with proper understanding of the nature and consequences of what is proposed,'* (Medical Research Council quoted in The College of Radiographers 1989). The use of the terms **valid consent** and **informed consent**, usually without definition, and frequently interchangeable, is indicative of the lack of consensus on the topic. No attempt is made here to define informed consent. Rather, it is discussed in the context of writing an acceptable PIS with the aim of helping researchers to obtain consent from potential participants in an ethically valid manner.

Figure 7.1 shows the breakdown of the whole concept into its two different parts: information and consent. It is helpful to look at these separately.

Informational elements

These are concerned with:

- *Disclosing to the potential participant all the information that they need to have to make up their mind about whether or not they wish to take part in your study*
- *Ensuring that the information is disclosed in such a way that enables the potential participant to fully understand what it is they are consenting to.*

The ideal way of obtaining informed consent is undocumented, probably because of the influence of individuality on the procedure.

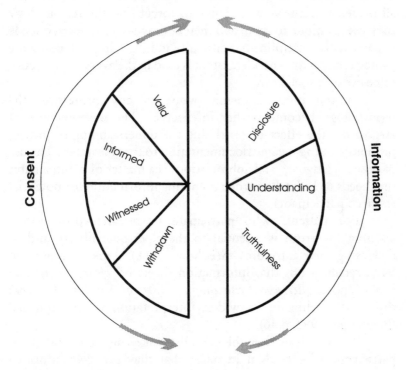

Figure 7.1 Informed consent: the two equal halves

Remember that one duty of the research is to tell the truth. Failure to tell the truth includes:

- *Under-disclosure*
- *Non-disclosure*
- *Disclosure that is unintelligible.*

The potential for unintelligible disclosure is great since, '*many doctors seem unaware how unintelligible medical terminology is to non-medical persons*,' (Robinson 1991, p.43). Not only doctors but all professionals have a tendency to forget that the terminology they use is unique to them and their colleagues. Anybody, outside of a particular discipline has difficulty in fully comprehending the profession specific knowledge that is used in the every-day practice of health and social care.

In the more academic work of any profession the terminology becomes rather intellectual. The increased use of **jargon** has the effect of restricting the understanding of project proposals and associated documentation to the researcher. The use of obscure language and abbreviations is a matter of habit; a habit that needs to be broken when preparing information for potential research participants.

For patients who participate in research programmes learning the truth is essential to their personal liberty and to increasing their autonomy (Seedhouse 1988). A recent report on REC recommends that information sheets be '*clear, concise and honest*' and '*explicit about risk and insurance cover in case of injury*'; thus truth telling in its widest interpretation is accomplished (Neuberger 1992, p.46).

The words used on the PIS must make sense to the potential participant who reads it in order that they can give informed consent. Examples of words that could be misunderstood, or not understood at all, and their suggested replacements are:

> *Seeds to be replaced by* **pellets**
>
> *Arm (of a trial) to be replaced by* **section**
>
> *Active to be replaced by* **known to work**
>
> *Resected to be replaced by* **removed**
>
> **Women like you** *to be replaced by* **patients with your condition**

Very technical terms are not appropriate on a PIS and you may need to rewrite the sentence or phase to explain what you mean or to remove offending or patronising words. The list below gives some examples of words that a REC had asked to be removed from a number of different PIS:

- *Enzyme*
- *Protocol*
- *Synthesis*
- *Animal studies*
- *Cell membrane.*

Potential participants may have a limited understanding of complex concepts associated with scientific studies. Researchers need to recognise this and to write in a clear and non-patronising way about the study. The finished PIS should:

- *Fully disclose all the details of the study*
- *Be written in a comprehensible, readable manner.*

Points that need addressing on the PIS include:

- *The continuation of the participants legal rights*
- *Other rights of the participants e.g. the right to withdraw at any time*
- *Matters of confidentiality and anonymity*
- *Risks and benefits of any interventions*
- *Any extra tests the participant may have to have, or additional journeys to the research setting, as the result of their participation*
- *Who is doing the study and how they can be contacted.*

Consent elements

The previous section discussed the rights of research participants to full information about any study they take part in. Of equal importance is the need to recognise that, in health and social care research, people may be asked to decide whether or not to participate in studies in circumstances that are far from ideal. Being ill, physically or psychologically, or being in a difficult family or social situation, increases our vulnerability to stress. In turn, this reduces our decision making capacity; we tend to reserve our strength for the absolutely necessary and give less attention to side issues.

At such times many people readily accept the wisdom of others, especially of experienced professionals and feel unable to actively seek out information in their interest. Others gain support from knowing as much as they can. They enter medical and other professional discussions about themselves with lists of questions. They feel comfortable enough to ask for time to think things over in their home environment, to discuss matters with their family and friends. Your potential research participants will be a mixture of both types of people, and with alterations in health and circumstances, people's behaviour may change.

Responsibility within research means having a sensitivity to this vulnerability of potential participants. Great care is needed during the process of obtaining consent and that care starts with the composition of the PIS. It is here that you can demonstrate to members of the REC, your honesty, and your understanding of the participants need for detailed and understandable information prior to consenting.

It was mentioned earlier that controversy surrounds the concept of informed consent. This not only relates to debating exactly 'what it is'; but also to whether, it is, at all times, necessary. It has been asked whether, in relation to randomised controlled trials, there are instances where ' "informed consent" (sic) is not necessary,' (Lancet 1990, p.847).

In addition, the design of certain studies may involve incomplete disclosure. For these the important question is, if the subject knew the retained information, would this alter their decision to consent (College of Psychiatrists 1990)? The ethical code of the College of Psychiatrists (1990), continues to say that a positive answer to this question means that the study should not be done. These are rare circumstances. The REC involved in scrutinising a study like that would need to judge such a research design, with very great regard for the autonomy of the participants and the potential benefits of the research.

Research on children may present problems with a full understanding of consenting and it may be children should never be participants in non-therapeutic research. Children and their parents are certainly seen as a vulnerable group by members of REC (Hammick 1993). Another view is that such research is permissible if the risks to the child are minimal and negligible, outweigh the benefits to the community as a whole and there is consent by proxy or a second party (Beauchamp & Childress 1983). Another vulnerable group of patients are those who are terminally ill. There is the danger of exploiting the wish of the patient to help others even when they know they cannot be helped themselves.

Witnessed consent is absolutely essential for certain participants. For example, the old and anyone with intellectual or cultural difficulties in speech or understanding,(Royal College of Physicians 1990, [ii]). Many consent forms require the signature of a witness to the consent procedure as standard but it is important to remember, once again, the patient's right to autonomy at this time. The researcher may need to make a moral judgement about whether inviting a witness is undermining that autonomy for some people. For others, who appear confused and are possibly willing to sign not having read the PIS, witnessed consent is essential to protect the research participant and the researcher.

Neuberger (1992, p.46) writes of the desirability of the presence of *'someone other than the researcher'* during the process of obtaining consent. You may be asked to act as a patient advocate or find yourself asking a colleague to act in this capacity for a potential participant for the study you are doing. In either situation, the rights of the potential participant are paramount.

7.4 Patient information sheets

This section looks at how to present the information about your study to potential participants in order that it meets the criteria previously discussed. Equally important, it is hoped that use of these guidelines will also mean that your local REC approves of any PIS you submit in an application for ethical scrutiny of a research project. Some ideas about the layout of a PIS are given, followed by an illustration of the information to include, using a PIS from a study which received ethical clearance.

Layout

If at all possible try to put all the necessary information onto one side of A4 paper. The PIS should be typed, with printing that is large enough to be easily read. Leave a space at the top to write the name of each person who agrees to be in your study. This confirms that it is information for them; a paper that they can keep to remind them of what they have consented to.

It is helpful for potential participants if you say exactly what it is they are about to read and head the PIS clearly e.g.

Participant Information Sheet

The reader immediately knows what it is they are reading and that it is supposed to give them information. Of course, it is unlikely that any researcher would give such a paper to a potential participant without some prior explanation. Nevertheless, a clear title to the PIS is helpful.

The first sentence is vital and it is here you need to remember that the person has not yet consented to be in your study. They are being given information to help them to make up their mind about whether they will participate, or not. This means they are not to be thanked for agreeing to participate but thanked for agreeing to read about your study! Acceptable words are:

> Thank you for agreeing to read this information which describes a project we are doing to find out what our patients know about radiotherapy and radiation.

Headings are useful throughout the sheet and the following are suggested ways in which you could breakdown the information you wish your participants to know before they give consent:

- *Background information*
- *Researchers responsible for the study*
- *The design of the study*
- *Potential side effects*
- *Potential benefits*
- *Confidentiality and anonymity*
- *Your rights as a participant*
- *Your involvement in the study.*

Different types of studies may demand different headings. Your role is to help the reader to fully understand the information on the sheet. Arranging all the necessary details about your study in a logical way is one way of doing this. The headings also act as a guide for you as you write the PIS.

A sample patient information sheet

In the following PIS the names of the investigators and the site of the research have all been anonymised for use as an example. The project for which it was written was called:

A qualitative study into knowledge and perceptions regarding radiotherapy and radiation in the patient population at St. Elsewheres NHS Trust.

The aims of the project were:

- *To acquire baseline information regarding what consented patients know about radiotherapy, where the information they have comes from, and how this influences their views about radiotherapy*
- *To identify language that is meaningful to patients regarding their own concepts of radiotherapy in order that patient information literature may better address issues of concern*
- *To identify the impact of media attention to radiotherapy and radiation use, on the consented radiotherapy patient.*

The PIS was as follows:

Patient Information Sheet

Thank you for agreeing to read this information which describes a project we are doing to find out what our patients know about radiotherapy and radiation.

Background information

- Many research projects have shown that patients find it helpful to have written information about their radiotherapy. We also know that the many different patients treated here have a variety of questions about radiotherapy and the effects of radiation. By doing this project we hope to learn how best to put together information to answer these question.

Researchers responsible for the study

Principal investigator: Ms A N Other, Senior Lecturer in
                                           Health Care Studies, University of
                                           the North. Tel. 1510 111 1234
                                           (direct line)

Co-investigators:	Dr B C Anon, Consultant Physician, St. Elsewheres NHS Trust. Tel. 1510 111 5678 or bleep 123
	Dr D E Further, Senior Registrar, St. Elsewheres NHS Trust. Tel. 1510 111 5678 or bleep 789

The design of the study

- For the project we want to interview 30 patients for no longer than one hour. The interview will be recorded on a small tape machine in order that we have an accurate record.

Potential benefits

- There are no direct benefits to you from participating in this project. We hope that our work will benefit patients in the future by helping us to give them the right sort of information about radiotherapy and radiation.

Confidentiality and anonymity

- All the recorded information will remain confidential to the research team and your name will not appear on any documentation. Each interview will be identified by number.

Your rights as participant

- Your right to take legal action in the event of any injury or damage arising out of this study will in no way be affected by giving consent to participate. If you decide not to take part, or agree and then change your mind and wish to withdraw, your current and future treatment will be unaffected by your decision.

Your involvement in the study

- Participation in the project will not mean you have to make any extra journeys to the Hospital. If you agree to participate we will arrange a date and time for the interview within one week of the start of your treatment. You should expect to spend a maximum of one hour longer at the Hospital on that day.

> • If you have any questions about this project, and if you agree to participate and wish to discuss any concerns you have related to radiotherapy after your interview, the researchers will be happy to talk to you. You can ask the staff to contact them on the telephone number given above.

Words and phrases

The example of a PIS given in the previous section uses words and phrases that are very specific to the type of research being done for that particular project. The topic of your project may be very different and will demand different words and possibly some different headings. If you are asked to scrutinise a number of PIS as a member of a REC you will see many different ones for lots of very different studies. This section looks at the type of information that should be included on every PIS. It also highlights some words and phrases linked with different research designs that can be misunderstood by people without some knowledge of research and health care work.

It is wise to include:

- *A statement about the participants legal rights*
- *An explanation about what will happen to those people who do not wish to participate, or withdraw after agreeing*
- *Who else might be told, with their permission, about the participation of the person in your study e.g. the hospital dietician, their general practitioner or hospital consultant*
- *The offer to send participants information of the findings of the study if they would like to know*
- *Statements about how confidentiality and anonymity will be ensured and who will have access to the data that is collected e.g. the research team and secretarial staff*

- *An explanation about the benefits, risks and side-effects, and to be honest about whether there will be any direct benefit to the participants*
- *Where there might be risk of injury to a participant they should be told about insurance cover*
- *Information about any financial benefits to the participants, and the researchers and organisation involved in the work.*

Other issues you should be very specific about include:

- *The time period over which the person will be participating. Use hours, days and weeks to convey this information. Try to be specific e.g.* **The canula will be in your arm for 48 hours** *and not to use phrases like* **We will give you five courses of treatment**
- *How the person has been selected to be asked to participate and how any further selection once they agree to take part will be made, this may mean explaining how the randomisation for a double blind clinical trial will be done. The patient has the right to know that randomisation will mean that the intervention they have will not have been selected by either themselves or their health care practitioner.*

It is also helpful to your potential participant if you choose words and phrases that they can understand, and do this without being patronising. Not always an easy task but, with attention to this, your PIS will be readable and will encourage the potential participant to freely give, or not give, informed consent. It is also a good idea to use the same words for describing the same thing. For example don't use **subject** and **participant** to describe the people who you will collect data from and select either **study** or **project** to describe the work you are doing.

Examples of increasing the **readability** are replacing:

- *Intravenous infusion with drip*
- *Subcutaneous injection with just under the skin*
- *Body image with how people see themselves.*

The previous sections have indicated the importance of being concise, truthful, using plain words and phrases that allow the reader to reach a full understanding of what you are telling them about your study. Writing a PIS for a study using people is a fundamental part of the research process; it is essential preparation for the task of accruing participants and collecting data. It will need to be included, probably as an appendix, in any application you make to your local REC for ethical clearance of the study. The way it is written, the language used and information included, is one way that the REC can form an opinion about your approach to research using people.

Applying some of the principles discussed in this chapter will help to make that task more straightforward. Using the REW you can carry out a self-scrutiny of what you are compiling. It is your responsibility to assemble the information to enable potential participants to genuinely give informed consent to becoming part of your research. In this way the research work reaches the professional standards that health care practitioners seek to maintain in their routine clinical work.

References

Anonymous (1990) *Medical ethics: should medicine turn the other cheek?* Lancet **336**: 846-7

Association of the British Pharmaceutical Industry (ABPI) (1990) *Guidelines for research ethics committees considering studies in healthy volunteers by pharmaceutical companies.* ABPI, London

Beauchamp T L & Childress J F (1983) *Principles of biomedical ethics.* 2nd Edn. Oxford University Press, New York

British Association of Occupational Therapists (1990) i. *Code of Professional Conduct.* College of Occupational Therapists, London

British Association of Occupational Therapists (1990) ii Occupational therapy research: how to do it. *Ethical Considerations.* College of Occupational Therapists, London

British Sociological Association (1993) *Statement of ethical practice*

Bryman A (1989). *Research methods and organisational studies.* Unwin Hyman Ltd, London

Buttigieg M, Meek R, Naish J & Burke E (undated) *An Introductory Guide to Research for Health Visitors and School Nurses.* Health Visitors Association, London

Clarke M, Kurinczuk J J for the Committee of Heads of Academic Departments of Public Health Medicine (1992) Health service research: a case of need or special pleading. *Br Med J* **304**: 1 675-6

College of Psychiatrists (1990) Guidelines for research ethics committees on psychiatric research involving human subjects. *Psych Bull* **14**: 48-61

College of Radiographers (1989) *Ethics and research projects.* College of Radiographers, London

College of Radiographers (1994) *A Strategy for Research.* College of Radiographers, London

Allen R E (Ed) (1990) *Concise Oxford Dictionary.* Clarendon Press, London

Denham M J, Foster A & Tyrrell D A J (1979) Work of a district ethical committee. *Br Med J* **2**: 1042-5

Department of Health (1991) *Local Research Ethics Committees.* HMSO, London

Department of Health (1992) *The Health of the Nation.* HMSO, London

Dickenson J A (1991) Getting help for research: the RACGP research committees. *Aust Fam Physician* **20** (11): 1659-62

Duerden B I, Reid T M S, Jewsbury J M & Turk D C (1987) *A New Short Textbook of Microbial and Parasitic Infection.* Edward Arnold, London

Ghazi F & Cook S (1993) Monitoring research in a nursing college. *Nurs Stan* August, 7 (47): 27-30

Gilbert C, Fulford K W M & Parker C (1989) Diversity in the practice of district ethics committees. *Br Med J* 299: 1437-9

Gilbert Foster C (1991) Ethics committees and health services research (letter). *J Pub Health Med* 13 (3): 230

Gilber Foster G C (1992) Research ethics committees – focus for the future. *Health Direct* **April/May,11**

Gillet G (1990) NZ medicine after Cartwright. *Br Med J* 300: 893-4

Ginzler M, Davies J, McPherson K & Black N (1990) Ethics committees and health services research. *J Pub Health Med* **12** (3/4): 190-6

Gould D (1987) *Infection and Patient Care, A Guide for Nurses.* Heinemann Medical Books, London

Halnan K (ed) (1980) *The Treatment of Cancer.* Chapman and Hall, London

Hammick M (1993) *Ethical Scrutiny Process and Debate, a case study of research ethics committee.* MSc Research dissertation, University of Southampton

Hancock B (1994) Your secrets are safe with us. *Nurs Stand* **8 (49)**: 44-45

Hunt G (1992) Nursing and Ethics Committees. *Ethics Forum 4.* National Centre for Nursing & Midwifery Ethics

King's Fund (1988) *The Nation's Health, a strategy for the 1990's.* Report from an independent multidisciplinary committee

Levine R J (1989) Institutional review boards Britain should consider the US example of more controlled ethics committees. *Br Med J* **298**: 1268-9

Lock S (1990) Monitoring research ethics committees. *Br Med J* 300: 61-2

MandellG L, Douglas R G & Bennett J E (1985) *Principles and Practice of Infectious Diseases.* 2nd Edn. John Wiley & Sons Ltd, New York

Neuberger J (1992) *Ethics and Health Care, the role of research ethics committees in the United Kingdom.* Research Report **13**, King's Fund Institute, London

Northern Regional Health Authority Working Group in Current Medical/Ethical problems, (1978) Report. *Lancet*1: 87-89

Nott P N & Steel E A (1988) Scrutinising research ethics committees (letter). *Br Med J* 297: 1333

Partridge C (1984) *Guidelines on ethics related to research in physiotherapy.* Centre for Physiotherapy Research

Popkin R H & Stroll A (1986) *Philosophy.* 2nd Edn. Made Simple Books, Butterworth-Heinemann Ltd, Oxford

Reason P & Rowan J (Eds) (1981) *Human Inquiry A Sourcebook of New Paradigm Research.* John Wiley & Sons Ltd, Chichester

Reason P (1981) Methodological approaches to social sciences by Ian Mitroff and Ralph Kilmann: an appreciation in Reason P & Rowan J (Eds) *Human Inquiry A Sourcebook of New Paradigm Research.* John Wiley & Sons Ltd, Chichester

Rowan J (1981) The subjective side of science by Ian Mitroff: an appreciation in Reason P and Rowan J (eds) *Human Inquiry A Sourcebook of New Paradigm Research.* John Wiley & Sons Ltd, Chichester

Robinson Sir K (1991) The Layman's Role in a Research Ethics Committee. *J Roy Coll Phys* 25: (1) 43

Royal College of Nursing Research Advisory Group (1993) *Ethics Related to Research in Nursing.* Scutari Press, Middlesex

Royal College of Physicians (1990) (i) *Research involving patients.* Royal College of Physicians, London

Royal College of Physicians (1990) (ii) *Guidelines on the practice of ethics committees in medical research involving human subjects.* (2nd Edn). Royal College of Physicians, London

Schrock R (1991) Moral issues in nursing research in Cormack D F S (Ed) *The nursing process in research.* 2nd Edn. Blackwell Scientific Publications, Oxford

Seedhouse D (1988) *Ethics the heart of health care.* John Wiley & Sons Ltd, Chichester

Seedhouse D & Lovett L (1992) *Practical Medical Ethics.* John Wiley & Sons Ltd, Chichester

Thompson I E, French K, Melia K M, Boyd K M, Templeton A A & Potter B (1981) Research ethical committtees in Scotland. *Br Med J* 282: 718-20

Thompson I E, Melia K M & Boyd K M (1988) *Nursing Ethics.* 2nd Edn. Churchill Livingstone, London

Von Wright G H (1978) Two traditions in Bynner J & Stribley K M (Eds) *Social research: principles and procedures.* Longman Group, London

Warnock M (1988) A national ethics committee To meet the growing demand for candour. *Br Med J* **297**: 1626-7

Waters W E & Cliff K S (1983) *Community medicine, a textbook for nurses and health visitors.* Croon Helm, Kent

Watson R (1969) *Edwin Chadwick Poor Law and Public Health.* Longman Group Ltd, London

World Medical Assembly (1964, 1975, 1983, 1989) *Declaration of Helsinki.* World Medical Association

Further reading and resources

Books

Beauchamp T L & Childress J F(1994) *Principles of Biomedical Ethics*. 4th Edn. Oxford University Press, New York
British Medical Association (1993) *Medical Ethics Today: Its Practice and Philosophy*. BMJ Publishing Group, London
Seedhouse D (1988) *Ethics The Heart of Health Care*. John Wiley & Sons Ltd, Chichester
Seedhouse D& Lovett L(1992) *Practical Medical Ethics*. John Wiley & Sons Ltd, Chichester
Cormack D F S[Ed] (1984) *The Nursing Process in Research*. 2nd Edn. Blackwell Scientific Publications, Oxford

Professional publications and codes of practice related to research ethics

British Association of Occupational Therapists (1990) *Code of Professional Conduct*. College of Occupational Therapists, London
British Sociological Association (1993) *Statement of Ethical Practice*.
Buttigieg M, Meek R, Naish J & Burke E (undated) *An Introductory Guide to Research for Health Visitors and School Nurses*. Health Visitors Association, London
College of Psychiatrists (1990) Guidelines for research ethics committees on psychiatric research involving human subjects. *Psych Bull* **14**: 48-61
College of Radiographers (1989) *Ethics and research projects*. College of Radiographers, London
Partridge C (1984) *Guidelines on Ethics Related to Research in Physiotherapy*. Centre for Physiotherapy Research, London

Royal College of Nursing Research Advisory Group (1993) *Ethics Related to Research in Nursing.* Scutari Press, MiddlesexRoyal College of Physicians (1990) *Research Involving Patients.* Royal College of Physicians, London

Royal College of Physicians (1990) *Guidelines on the practice of ethics committees in medical research involving human subjects.* Royal College of Physicians, London

Other useful publications

Department of Health (1991) *Local Research Ethics Committees.* HMSO, London

Medical Research Council Working Party on Research on Children (1991) *The Ethical Conduct of Research on Children.* The Medical Research Council, London

Medical Research Council Working Party on Ethical Aspects of AIDS Vaccine Trials (1991) *The Ethical Aspects of AIDS Vaccine Trials.* The Medical Research Council, London

Medical Research Council Working Party on Research On The Mentally Incapacitated (1991) *The Ethical Conduct Of Research On The Mentally Incapacitated.* The Medical Research Council, London

Neuberger J (1992) *Ethics and Health Care, the role of research ethics committees in the United Kingdom.* Research Report **13**, Kings Fund Institute, London

Glossary

Beneficence   A principle of ethical behaviour which means to do good in an active and positive manner.

Deotonology   The study of duty.

Double blind clinical trial   Research designed to ensure that neither the participants, who may receive one of two or more alternative interventions, or the researcher measuring the results of any intervention, knows which participants receive which intervention.

Empirical   This usually refers to evidence or data which is based on the results of an experiment or observation; in contrast to theoretical reasoning.

Ethnographic   A research style that recognises the human nature of the participants. Data is analysed within the cultural context from which it was collected.

Interpreter	In this context the word is used to mean someone who translates written and spoken information for people without English as a first language during the process of giving informed consent. It is recognised that this is best done by professional interpreters. However, such people are not always available in health and social care settings and staff with foreign language skills may be asked to substitute.
Interviews	A face-to-face encounter between the researcher and participant in which data is collected for the purpose of analysis, the depth of relationship between the interviewee and interviewer varies with interview type.
structured interviews	are those where the researcher sets the questions in advance and only these questions are used in the interview(s). The interviewer would rarely build a relationship with the research participant.
semi-structured interviews	Are those where the researcher has a set of themes to cover and initiates a conversation with the participant on these. At the same time the participant is allowed to wander from the theme and thus to contribute

views on issues not necessarily covered by the original themes. Sometimes these are called **a conversation with a purpose.** Building rapport with the interviewee is essential to the success of the interview.

unstructured interviews

are those where the researcher engages in very casual conversation with participant in order to have an exchange of ideas and views on a set topic. The resulting dialogue that follows very much takes the direction dictated by the participant and, inevitably, a relationship develops between the interviewee and interviewer.

Paradigm

A way of seeing things or a model for a particular discipline that is suggestive of the scope of the discipline, and the means of investigating practice within the discipline. Often used to imply that the model referred to is the ideal, or of major influence.

Patient advocate

A member of the patient's family, or a friend, or a member of the health care team who acts on behalf of the patient and in the best interests of the patient. Especially in situations where decisions may need to be made and the patient's present situation or state of health may mean that they are not fully able to make coherent and rational decisions alone. In these circumstances some help and explanation by someone who looks at the issues involved from their point of view is sought.

Performance status

A measurement of the patient's general condition on a spectrum from ability to carry on with normal activities, through items such as 'caring for self, unable to work' and 'severely disabled, needs hospital care', to dead. Examples of these include the Swiss and Karnofsky Scales (Halnan 1982).

Phenomeno-logical

A research style that considers knowledge to be inherently subjective, personal, societal and cultural. The experiences of the participants are transformed into data for analysis with sympathy for context and relationships.

Positivistic

A research style that is traditional, objective and deals with measurable data. It claims to deal in facts in a value-free environment.

Quality Adjusted Life Years (QALYs) Estimates of survival corrected for quality of life by multiplying life expectancy data by **quality of life** values for different groups of patients.

Quality of life values Outcomes of research which consider the quality of life of the patient that results from an intervention in contrast to simply measuring any extension of life in months and years.

Qualitative research Research strategies which seek to capture data from the perspective of the research participants and to investigate participants in depth; has many synonyms including fieldwork, ethnomethodological and interpretive.

Quantitative research Research strategies generating large amounts of data which are then analysed using appropriate statistical methods.

Reliability The consistency/stability of any measurement tool; external reliability relates to consistency over time and internal reliability to consistency within internal groups of research participants.

Sampling frame   The complete population from
                       which a sample is selected for
                       research purposes.

Self-reporting   Used to gather data from research
diary cards   participants over a set period of
                       time where that data is best
                       collected   by   asking   the
                       participant to record set items
                       themselves on a form designed
                       for that purpose.

Statistical   Measures of this are related to the
significance   confidence we can have that the
                       findings about a sample of a
                       population can be applied to the
                       complete population.

Survival   Most   normally,   survival   is
statistics   measured as either **morbidity**
                       which is indicative of the amount
                       of disease present or **mortality**
                       which indicates the death rate.

Validity   This relates to whether a measure
                       is related to whatever it claims to
                       measure; there are many types of
                       validity   e.g.   face   validity,
                       criterion validity and construct
                       validity (for more detail see
                       Bryman 1989, and others).

Variables   Characteristics   of   research
                       participants   which   show
                       difference across the selected
                       sample.

Abbreviations and acronyms

ABPI	Association of the British Pharmaceutical Industry
DHA	District Health Authority
DOH	Department of Health
NHS	National Health Service
NEC	National Ethics Committee
PIS	Patient Information Sheet(s)
PLI	Product Liability Insurance
PSMs	Professions Supplementary to Medicine
QALYs	Quality Adjusted Life Years
R&D	Research and Development
REC	Research Ethics Committee(s)
REW	Research Ethics Wheel
SRC	Scientific Review Committee(s)
WMA	World Medical Assembly

Index